MAGNESIUM

The Missing Mineral

Discover the vital role Magnesium plays in your health

DR. JAMES DINICOLANTONIO

DR. BARB WOEGERER, ND

2024

DISCLAIMER

Legal & Disclaimer

The information contained in this book is not designed to replace or take the place of any form of medicine or professional medical advice. The information in this book has been provided for educational purposes only.

The information contained in this book has been compiled from sources deemed reliable, and it is accurate to the best of the authors' knowledge; however, the authors cannot guarantee its accuracy and validity and cannot be held liable for any errors or omissions. Changes are periodically made to this book. You must consult your doctor or get professional medical advice before using any of the suggested remedies, techniques, or information in this book.

Upon using the information contained in this book, you agree to hold harmless the authors and publisher from and against any damages, costs, and expenses, including any legal fees potentially resulting from the application of any of the information provided by this guide. This disclaimer applies to any damages or injury caused by the use and application, whether directly or indirectly, of any advice or information presented, whether for breach of contract, tort, negligence, personal injury, criminal intent, or under any other cause of action.

You agree to accept all risks of using the information presented inside this book. You need to consult a professional medical practitioner in order to ensure you are both able and healthy enough to participate in this program.

Jacket design by James DiNicolantonio and Barb Woegerer.

Table of Contents

About the Authors

Dr. James DiNicolantonio

As a cardiovascular research scientist and Doctor of Pharmacy, Dr. James J. DiNicolantonio has spent years researching nutrition. A well-respected and internationally known scientist and expert on health and nutrition, he has contributed extensively to health policy and medical literature. Dr. DiNicolantonio is the author of 9 best-selling health books, The Salt Fix, 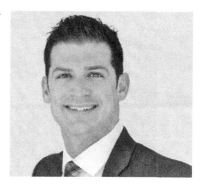 Superfuel, The Longevity Solution, The Immunity Fix, The Mineral Fix, WIN, The Obesity Fix, The Collagen Cure and The Blood Sugar Fix. His website is www.drjamesdinic.com. You can follow Dr. DiNicolantonio on Twitter and Instagram at @drjamesdinic and Facebook at Dr. James DiNicolantonio. You can find the magnesium and all the supplements Dr. James DiNicolantonio takes by going to the Fullscript link in his Instagram bio @drjamesdinic.

Dr. Barb Woegerer, ND

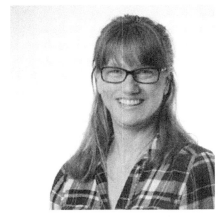

Dr. Barb Woegerer is a licensed Naturopathic Doctor, speaker, and content creator based in Ontario, Canada. With a wealth of experience in health and wellness, she has made it her mission to empower individuals to take charge of their well-being through evidence-based therapies. Dr. Barb is particularly passionate about the critical role magnesium plays in overall health, dedicating extensive time to researching and advocating for greater awareness of this essential mineral. Her commitment to helping others understand and address the importance of magnesium is a driving force behind her work. To learn more, you can follow her on Instagram at @drbarbwoegerer and on Facebook at Dr. Barb Woegerer, Naturopathic Doctor. You can visit her website at https://www.barbwoegerer.com.

To Michael Madonik, MD—my heartfelt thanks for your unwavering support.

- Dr. Barb Woegerer, ND

Introduction

Magnesium is an essential mineral, meaning we must get it from our diet. Magnesium is also the seventh most abundant element in the Earth's crust and the second most common positively charged electrolyte inside our cells (second only to potassium).[1] Around 99% of all magnesium contained in the body can be found inside the cell, whereas only around 1% is found outside of the cell. The human body contains around 25 grams of magnesium with 90% being found in muscle and bone.

Magnesium is an elemental powerhouse with a rich history that unveils its crucial role in science and medicine. Understanding magnesium's historical timeline is essential. It provides us with the opportunity to understand its role in human health and how it has shaped medical interventions. Exploring magnesium's historical backdrop sheds light on its therapeutic potential and emphasizes its critical role as a fundamental component of human biology. Understanding this narrative will unveil the profound implications that magnesium holds for our health and well-being.

Magnesium is considered a key essential mineral crucial for optimal bodily function. Magnesium acts as a critical cofactor in more than 600 enzymatic reactions in the body.[2] It is involved in almost every major metabolic and biochemical process within the cell. This emphasizes its importance in sustaining health and vitality.

Originating from the discovery of magnesium carbonate, a region in Thessaly, Greece, known as Magnesia, the name "magnesium" carries historical weight. The utilization of magnesium in human medicine dates back to 1695 when Dr. Nehemiah Grew made a groundbreaking discovery. He identified magnesium sulfate ($MgSO_4$) as the key component of Epsom salt, derived from wells in Epsom, England. Epsom salt quickly gained popularity for its effectiveness in treating a wide range of ailments, everything from abdominal discomfort to muscle strains. Dr. Nehemiah Grew's exploration of the bitter mineral water from Epsom wells opened the door to creating solid magnesium sulfate, known today as "Epsom salts."[3]

Magnesium was recognized and identified as an element, symbolized as "Mg" in 1755 by Joseph Black. Then, in 1808, English chemist Sir Humphrey Davy made a significant breakthrough by isolating magnesium for the first time from magnesium oxide.[4] Despite magnesium salts being recognized in plants during the eighteenth century, their importance in animals was not fully understood until later.

In 1926, the significance of magnesium as an essential mineral came to light. Jehan Leroy's research showcased the essential nature of magnesium for sustaining life in mice. Their early studies involved giving mice diets low in magnesium, causing acute deficiency states.[5] By replenishing the mice with magnesium, researchers gained a clearer picture of how this mineral works in mammals. In 1934, Arthur Hirschfelder and Victor Haury identified the first documented case of "frank" magnesium deficiency in humans. However, it wasn't until later that scientists began to explore chronic magnesium deficiency, a condition more closely resembling the scenarios observed in humans.

In 1965, M.S. Seelig conducted a review of metabolic studies.[6] She found that to maintain balance and prevent magnesium loss from the body, individuals need about 6.9 mg of magnesium per kilogram of body weight.[6] For example, a person weighing 70 kg (154 lbs) would require approximately 483 mg of magnesium daily to stay in equilibrium. However, it wasn't until much later that researchers realized that healthy individuals could adapt to lower magnesium intakes. Around 180 mg per day was found to be sufficient for maintaining balance in optimal health conditions. Importantly, however, maintaining balance is not the same thing as getting an optimal intake. Indeed, many studies now indicate that getting around 6.9 mg of magnesium per kilogram (483 mg for an average person) is closer to an optimal intake than 180 mg per day.[1, 7]

There are more than 60 factors contributing to magnesium deficiency that have been identified. Subclinical, or marginal magnesium deficiency, can be tricky to recognize because it does not always present with any obvious symptoms. Unfortunately, it can lead to serious long term health problems like osteoporosis, hypertension, heart disease and more. Research indicates that around 15-20% of the population may be magnesium deficient based solely on blood levels. However, the actual number seems to be much higher (around 30-50%) when we consider better ways to test for magnesium deficiency.

This highlights the urgent need to address magnesium deficiency as it poses a widespread and pressing public health concern.

Unfortunately, since the 1970s, only a few have recognized the widespread issue of low magnesium intake in developed countries. If this deficiency persists, it can lead to various health issues affecting almost every system in the body. Dietary habits marked by low magnesium intake, high phosphate intake, high animal fat and sugar consumption contribute to magnesium loss. Additionally, medications like diuretics, laxatives, and antacids, as well as supplements such as calcium and vitamin D can also increase the risk of magnesium deficiency. Lifestyle factors like stress, alcohol consumption, excessive caffeine intake, and participation in endurance sports further compound the risk of magnesium loss.

As mentioned previously, one of the big challenges with marginal or subclinical magnesium deficiency is that it does not typically have obvious symptoms. In addition, it is very difficult to detect through standard blood tests because over 99% of magnesium is inside our cells and not in our blood. The consequences of low magnesium levels can take a long time to develop, making it difficult for doctors to pinpoint magnesium deficiency as the underlying issue for health problems. As a result, most individuals are unaware of the condition because it's rarely diagnosed unless they show clear symptoms.

The good news is that there is a growing awareness of subclinical magnesium deficiency happening. It underscores the importance of recognizing that even without visible symptoms, there could still be significant health risks. You may be seemingly thriving despite being magnesium deficient and then suddenly, out of nowhere, conditions like irregular heartbeats or fractures could show up. It's a reminder that sometimes, the most serious threats are the ones we can't see coming.

When your magnesium intake is low, you won't notice that your body is absorbing less calcium or that it is activating less vitamin D. It's hard to feel or notice when magnesium is being drawn from your bones due to a low magnesium diet, that is of course until you experience a bone fracture. However, fractures are often attributed to 'old age' or 'fall-related' rather than the true cause or root cause — fragile bones from magnesium deficiency. Imagine if your medical report pointed to 'magnesium deficiency-induced osteoporosis' instead of simply blaming age or falls. Unfortunately, physicians will then suggest taking more calcium and Vitamin D, which can actually make the magnesium deficiency worse.

However, subclinical magnesium deficiency is not just about long-term health risks. It can also lead to acute diseases. For instance, a lack of magnesium can weaken immune function, making viral or bacterial infections more severe and potentially fatal for vulnerable individuals. It is for this reason why a magnesium deficiency has been deemed the single largest health problem in our world today.

Magnesium research continues to thrive across various fields, spanning from basic sciences to pathology. A simple search of "Magnesium" in the PubMed Database returns an astonishing 120,000 entries, showcasing the extensive exploration surrounding this essential mineral. This vast collection of research underscores the ongoing quest to understand magnesium's impact on our health. With each study, we gain valuable insights into magnesium's impacts on human health, reaffirming its essential status in our pursuit for wellness.

Our commitment lies in emphasizing the crucial importance of magnesium and its profound impact on human health. As you journey through the pages of this book, our aim is to provide you with insights and knowledge that will deepen your appreciation for the critical role magnesium plays in maintaining optimal health. Together, let's pave the way for a journey toward wellness and vitality. Magnesium is not just a mineral; it is our partner in health.

Chapter 1: Subclinical Magnesium Deficiency

Subclinical magnesium deficiency is a common, yet under-recognized problem throughout the world. Understanding the importance of magnesium is vital. Given its role in facilitating over 600 enzymatic reactions within the human body, maintaining adequate levels of magnesium is essential.[2, 8] The majority of the body's vital enzymes rely on magnesium for their proper function. About 90% of our total magnesium is found in the muscles and bones, with roughly 27% in muscles and 63% in bones.[9] Most of this magnesium is tied up, with only 10% available for immediate use.[9] Within the bloodstream, approximately 32% of magnesium binds to a protein known as albumin, while the remaining 55% circulates freely.[9]

Magnesium plays several important roles in the body. Some of the main functions include maintaining the right balance of certain minerals inside cells, keeping sodium and calcium low, and keeping potassium high. Magnesium also supports the structure of cells and tissues, helps produce energy in the cells' powerhouses (mitochondria), and contributes to the synthesis and integrity of DNA, RNA, and proteins.[10, 11]

The kidneys play a key role in regulating magnesium levels in the body, getting rid of excess magnesium through urine when there's too much, and reducing it to just a small amount when levels are low.[10] However, even with this regulation in place, the body can pull magnesium from the bones, muscles, and organs to keep blood magnesium levels normal when intake is insufficient.[12, 13] What this essentially means is that having a normal magnesium level in the blood does not actually rule out magnesium deficiency.

Magnesium deficiency can contribute to a range of health issues, spanning from bone and heart issues to brain disorders and metabolic complications. Environmental factors play a significant role in micronutrient deficiencies. Soil contamination with heavy metals poses a threat to plant growth and nutrient uptake.[14] Additionally, a decrease in minerals in the soil contributes to the depletion of minerals in plants and the animals that eat them.[14] As soil erodes, it strips away the fertile top layer that contains essential minerals necessary for plant growth and health. This process reduces the availability of minerals like magnesium, calcium, potassium, and others in the soil, making it more challenging for plants to absorb these nutrients. In the past, there was a greater focus and emphasis on the mineral content of soil and water, which is vital for health. However, this significance has unfortunately been forgotten over time.[15] Additionally, processed foods, which constitute a significant portion of our diet, undergo refining and manufacturing processes that lead to a loss of magnesium content.[16] Thus, if we want to prevent chronic diseases, we must shift our focus from exclusively treating acute illnesses to addressing the actual root causes of chronic conditions, one of them being magnesium deficiency.

To understand deficiencies, it's essential to differentiate between two distinct types: frank deficiency and subclinical deficiency. Frank deficiencies have clear symptoms such as scurvy from a lack of vitamin C or goiter from iodine deficiency. Subclinical deficiencies occur without obvious signs but can still affect physiological, cellular and/or biochemical functions. Subclinical deficiencies are particularly worrisome as they are challenging to detect and can lead to various chronic diseases. While both types of deficiencies have negative health impacts, frank deficiencies show obvious symptoms, whereas subclinical deficiencies have subtle but harmful effects. Research suggests that subclinical magnesium deficiency is widespread and a major contributor to chronic diseases and premature death worldwide, warranting attention as a major public health crisis.[1, 17-19]

Magnesium Intake

The body's homeostatic mechanisms to maintain magnesium balance were developed a long time ago, back when our ancestors were hunter-gatherers. Research into their diet shows they consumed around 600 mg of magnesium daily, much more than what most people consume today. Despite the passage of time, our body's natural balance and genetic makeup remain similar to those of our Paleolithic ancestors, suggesting that our metabolism functions best with a higher magnesium intake.[9]

In modern developed nations, the average daily magnesium intake is just over 4 mg per kilogram of body weight (around 280 mg for a 70 kg adult).[20] This low level of intake is concerning, especially considering that more than a quarter of both obese and non-obese children do not get enough magnesium in their diets.[21] This points to a concerning trend where children may be consuming too many calories but not enough essential nutrients (sometimes referred to as high calorie malnutrition). It has been argued that while a typical Western diet might prevent frank magnesium deficiency, it's unlikely to maintain optimal magnesium levels needed for reducing the risk of conditions like heart disease and osteoporosis. Several studies have shown that supplementing with at least 300 mg of magnesium daily can get magnesium levels in the blood to a more optimal range.[9] In essence, for many individuals, an extra 300 mg of magnesium each day may be needed to lower the risk of developing numerous chronic diseases. The recommended daily allowance (RDA) for magnesium falls between 310 mg and 420 mg per day for most individuals. Merely meeting this requirement may prevent frank magnesium deficiency. However, to achieve optimal health and longevity, it's likely that more magnesium than the recommended daily allowance (RDA) is needed.

It's important to note that many individuals worldwide are not getting enough magnesium in their diets, even falling short of the Recommended Dietary Allowance (RDA). The Recommended Dietary Allowance (RDA) measures the average daily intake of a nutrient needed to meet the nutritional requirements of most healthy individuals in a specific age and gender group. For example, in Taiwan, men and women typically consume only 68% to 70% of the recommended dietary magnesium intake.[22] While this might be enough to avoid severe magnesium deficiency, it may not be sufficient enough to lower the risk of conditions like diabetes, especially among the elderly.[22] Similarly, in Japan, magnesium intake among individuals aged 15 to 49 is below the recommended dietary allowance levels.[23] In the United States, nearly half of the population does not meet the recommended magnesium intake from food alone.[24] The US Department of Agriculture reports that women consume an average of 228 mg per day of magnesium, while men consume an average of 323 mg per day. This suggests that a significant number of people may be at risk for magnesium deficiency, particularly if they have other health conditions or take certain medications that further deplete magnesium levels.[12] Recent research further indicates that 50% of Americans consume less than the Estimated Average Requirement (EAR) for magnesium, with some age groups consuming notably lower amounts.[25] The Estimated Average Requirement (EAR) is a benchmark value used in dietary assessments and planning to ensure that the nutritional needs of most people in a specific population are met.

Researchers collected the daily dietary intake of 34 men and women for a year. They found that on average men consumed about 323 mg of magnesium per day, while women had about 234 mg per day. This is roughly 4 mg per kilogram of body weight. Surprisingly, despite this intake, most people were actually in a negative magnesium balance (-32 mg/day for men and -25 mg/day for women)[26]. Many women, about 75%, were not even meeting the recommended daily allowance of 300 mg per day. Given that the typical magnesium intake in the USA is approximately 228 mg per day for women and 266 mg per day for men[17], a significant portion of Americans are at risk of negative magnesium balance. In fact, it was stated that "Only American diets containing more than 3000 kcal per day may provide 300 mg or more of magnesium."[26] A long-term study lasting 50 weeks showed that to maintain a positive magnesium balance, an intake of between 180 mg and 320 mg of magnesium per day is necessary.[27] Moreover, fiber binds magnesium, reducing its absorption. Individuals on high fiber diets consuming 322 mg of magnesium per day have been noted to have negative magnesium balance.[28] Since many individuals are consuming below 320 mg of magnesium per day, this poses a major health threat.

Around the globe, similar issues with inadequate magnesium intake persist. In Germany, for instance, women only get about 200 mg and men about 250 mg of magnesium per day.[9, 29] In Kiev, researchers found that 780 men aged 20-59 were not getting enough magnesium in their diets. The researchers also found a correlation between the low magnesium intake from food and the prevalence of risk factors for ischemic heart disease, including hyperlipoproteinemia, high blood pressure, and body weight.[30] Women, in particular, tend to exhibit lower levels of magnesium intake compared to men. Studies in France showed that a significant portion of the population, especially women, were not getting enough magnesium. Magnesium deficiency during pregnancy can lead to consequences for both the mother and child, with potential effects such as Sudden Infant Death Syndrome (SIDS).[31] Finally, In Southern France, magnesium intake among elderly individuals aged 70 years or older was found to be below the recommended dietary allowance.[32]

Magnesium Deficiency

Hypomagnesemia, or low magnesium levels, is quite common in the medical world. Magnesium deficiency often goes unnoticed because clinicians do not usually evaluate for magnesium levels. Unfortunately, many times these clinicians do not fully recognize the various health conditions that could result from too little or too much magnesium in the body.[33]

In developed countries, older studies estimated that about 15% to 20% of the population may have a marginal magnesium deficit.[20] More recent research suggests that between 10% and 30% of individuals could actually have a subclinical magnesium deficiency, based on low levels of magnesium in their blood (<0.80 mmol/L).[25] A systematic review of 37 articles revealed that magnesium deficiency could be a potential public health issue among older adults.[34]

Interestingly, even when blood tests show normal magnesium levels, magnesium deficiency can still be present.[11] Magnesium deficiency was shown in 84% of postmenopausal women diagnosed with osteoporosis.[35] They were diagnosed by low magnesium trabecular bone content and the Thoren's magnesium load test. In addition, low levels of magnesium were also found in 75% of patients with poorly controlled type 2 diabetes.[36] Among elderly individuals, 20% were found to have low magnesium and potassium levels in their red blood cells.[37]

With these statistics, it's important to note that the range considered normal for magnesium levels in the blood doesn't tell us the whole story. When magnesium levels in the blood are at the lower end of what's considered normal, this likely suggests marginal magnesium deficiency.[1, 25] This indicates that relying solely on blood tests to assess magnesium levels is not an accurate reflection of magnesium status in the body. Muscle biopsy is also a more accurate indicator of the body's magnesium content.[38]

In line with this, another research study revealed the discrepancy between magnesium levels in the blood and those in the body's tissues. The study found that even though the blood levels of potassium (K) and magnesium (Mg) in patients undergoing long-term treatment for hypertension or heart disease appeared normal, about half of them had reduced levels of magnesium and potassium in their muscles.[39] Therefore, evaluating

18

potassium and magnesium levels during diuretic treatment should preferentially involve checking the levels in the tissues. A muscle biopsy, a more reliable method, may better reveal these deficiencies. But there is good news…and that is that oral supplementation of magnesium was found to be effective in restoring normal potassium and magnesium levels.[39]

In critical medical settings, such as postoperative recovery units and medical intensive care units (ICUs), studies have revealed alarming rates of magnesium deficiency among patients. Among postoperative patients, 36.5% showed low ionized magnesium levels in their red blood cells (ionized magnesium is the active unbound form),[40] while a staggering 65% of ICU patients were found to have low magnesium levels in the blood.[41] This prevalence of low magnesium levels in critically ill patients underscores the potential risks associated with magnesium deficiency, including hypocalcemia (low blood calcium), hypokalemia (low blood potassium), heart rhythm disturbances and other symptoms.[41] In addition, it was noted that hypomagnesemia (low magnesium levels) detected in acutely ill medical patients upon admission has been linked to increased mortality rates for both ward and medical ICU patients.[42]

Magnesium depletion is also prevalent among ICU patients, with approximately half experiencing this deficiency.[43] Alarmingly, more than 50% of hospitalized patients with various medical conditions, including hypertension, coronary artery disease, cerebrovascular events, gastrointestinal issues, or alcoholism, are likely to be magnesium-deficient based on intravenous retention rates exceeding 20%.[44] These findings highlight the critical importance of recognizing and addressing magnesium deficiency in clinical settings to improve patient outcomes and overall health.

A comprehensive review of 183 scientific studies spanning from 1990 to 2008 revealed an intriguing finding: many medical professionals subscribe to the notion that having 'normal' magnesium levels signifies the absence of deficiency. This perception may stem from the fact that laboratories typically highlight only abnormal results, potentially skewing the interpretation of 'normal' levels. It's important to be cautious about relying too much on 'normal' magnesium levels in the blood because it may lead to overlooking a magnesium deficiency. In addition, many physicians do not initiate requests to look at magnesium blood levels. This highlights a significant oversight by medical professionals regarding low magnesium levels in the blood. This is concerning because restoring deficient magnesium levels in patients is straightforward, safe, cost-effective, and can profoundly improve health outcomes.

When it comes to certain medications, patients may exhibit normal or elevated magnesium levels in the blood, even in the presence of magnesium depletion. For example, roughly 80% of patients with hypertension who took hydrochlorothiazide or a single non-diuretic drug for at least 6 months were found to be depleted in magnesium.[45] What's concerning is that despite this magnesium depletion, patients treated with hydrochlorothiazide often had normal or even high levels of magnesium in their blood. This highlights a significant issue: patients can have normal or higher magnesium levels in their blood even when their body lacks magnesium. Another study supported these findings by showing that thiazide diuretics cause magnesium depletion that cannot be detected by checking magnesium levels in the blood.[46] Additionally, there is a correlation between low magnesium levels in bones and increased magnesium retention after receiving an intravenous magnesium load, suggesting that magnesium is lost from bone during deficiency.[47] In fact, by the time we reach 50 years old we may have lost 50% of the magnesium from our bone.[29]

Strenuous physical activity is another factor to consider when discussing magnesium deficiency. After several weeks of intense physical activity, the level of magnesium in the blood may increase even though the magnesium levels in mononuclear cells are reduced.[48] The researchers noted that the decrease in magnesium levels in mononuclear cells indicates less magnesium stored in the body. This suggests that engaging in strenuous physical activity for just 6 to 12 weeks increases magnesium need and can lead to magnesium deficiency. Another study found that during a marathon, both blood and urine magnesium levels drop, suggesting increased magnesium need due to increased demand for magnesium in the skeletal muscles.[49]

When testing serum magnesium levels a normal serum magnesium level falls between 0.7–1 mmol/L.[50] However, optimal serum magnesium levels should be higher than 0.80 mmol/L.[50] Chronic latent magnesium deficiency is when the serum magnesium concentration ranges from 0.75 to 0.849 mmol/L, which falls within the normal reference interval, with a positive magnesium load test indicating magnesium deficiency.[19]

Overall, abnormalities in serum magnesium may be the most commonly missed electrolyte abnormality in clinical practice, with a reported incidence ranging from 12.5% to 20% in routine tests.[51] Additionally, someone can have a normal total magnesium level in the blood but low ionic magnesium (which is the active form) in blood or red blood cells.[40] Thus, we believe that ionic magnesium levels should also be measured (in blood and red blood cells) to assess magnesium status.

'Normal' Serum Magnesium Levels[1] 0.75–0.95 mmol/L[25]

▶ A serum magnesium < 0.82 mmol/L (< 2.0 mg/dL) with a 24-hour urinary magnesium excretion of 40–80 mg/day is highly suggestive of magnesium deficiency.[25]

▶ One group of experts has recommended magnesium supplementation in subjects experiencing symptoms that reflect magnesium deficiency if the serum level is below 0.9 mmol/L, with levels less than 0.8 mmol/L necessitating magnesium.[52]

▶ Serum magnesium levels above 0.95 mmol/L may indicate hypermagnesemia.

Maintaining a Positive Magnesium Balance

To maintain the right amount of magnesium in the body, it's a balance between how much we get from our diet and how much we lose. Our body absorbs about one-third of the magnesium we ingest, mainly in the small intestine. Thus, if we consume 300 mg of magnesium per day, around 100 mg should come out in the urine over 24 hours.[53] Our body regulates this balance by adjusting how much magnesium it holds onto or eliminates based on our intake.

A study involving 11 postmenopausal women aged 49–71 found that an intake of 107 mg per day of magnesium was not enough to maintain a positive magnesium balance.[54] In a placebo-controlled trial, women (aged 20 to 69) who consumed 205 mg and 376 mg of magnesium daily (from their omnivore and lacto-ovo vegetarian diets, respectively) were in negative magnesium balance. Even when they were supplemented with an additional 100 mg of magnesium they failed to achieve a positive or even neutral magnesium balance, despite showing increased magnesium excretion in their urine.[9,

55] This means that women might still be in a negative magnesium balance despite consuming between 305 mg and 476 mg of magnesium per day. In a more recent study with postmenopausal women, they found that a diet providing 399 milligrams of magnesium per 2000 calories was able to produce a positive magnesium balance.[56] However, a diet with only about 100 milligrams of magnesium per 2000 calories was not adequate.[56] Men with osteoporosis or psychoneurosis had a negative magnesium balance when consuming between 240 and 264 milligrams of magnesium daily.[57] What all of these findings show is that various factors like diet, stress, health conditions, and medications play a role in magnesium balance. These factors all increase magnesium requirements.

According to data from the National Health and Nutrition Examination Survey (NHANES), 64% of women aged 51–70, do not meet the estimated average requirement (EAR) for magnesium for their age group, which is 265 mg per day.[28] Their average magnesium intake was estimated at only 246 mg per day in 2001–2002 and even lower at 238 mg per day in 1999–2000. Mexican and African–American women in the same age group have even lower magnesium intakes, ranging from 150 mg to 185 mg per day, especially for those not using dietary supplements.[28] Therefore, this highlights that the elderly population are particularly vulnerable to magnesium deficiency because of low dietary intake and a higher likelihood of chronic diseases that can lead to magnesium deficiency. Additionally, as individuals age, their ability to absorb magnesium from the diet diminishes, primarily due to a decline in stomach acid production.

Causes of Magnesium Deficiency

There are many factors that can lead to a magnesium deficiency. Understanding the multitude of factors contributing to magnesium deficiency is crucial due to its pervasive impact on health. With at least 60 potential causes, ranging from dietary habits to underlying health conditions, medications, malabsorption issues, alcohol consumption, physical activity and more. Our modern lifestyles inadvertently chip away at our magnesium levels, leaving us vulnerable to a host of health issues. When we can recognize the diverse array of causes, it enables healthcare professionals and individuals alike to address and mitigate the risk of magnesium deficiency more effectively.

In the body, three important organs work together to keep magnesium levels balanced:

- The small and large intestines absorb magnesium from the food we eat.

- Bones, which serves as the body's main storage system for this mineral.

- Kidneys, control magnesium levels by releasing it into the urine or holding on to it.

Any disruption at any stage of this process can be a cause for magnesium deficiency.[58]

The following are some of the most common causes of magnesium deficiency that disrupt one or more of these stages.

Gastrointestinal Disorders

Individuals with conditions affecting the intestines or colon like Crohn's disease, Ulcerative Colitis, Irritable Bowel Syndrome, Gastroenteritis, Celiac disease, Ileostomy patients and others are more likely to experience magnesium deficiency. These conditions often involve inflammation and damage to the intestines, which can impair the absorption of magnesium.[10] Additionally, chronic diarrhea, common in Crohn's disease and Ulcerative Colitis, can lead to excessive loss of magnesium through the feces.

Low stomach acid, a condition known as hypochlorhydria, is increasingly recognized as a significant factor that contributes to magnesium deficiency.[59] In our modern society, the prevalence of low stomach acid is noteworthy. Stomach acid plays a crucial role in the absorption of magnesium from the food we consume. When stomach acid levels are low, as is the case with hypochlorhydria, the absorption of magnesium becomes compromised.[60] Magnesium requires an acidic environment in the stomach for optimal absorption. Without sufficient stomach acid, magnesium absorption is hindered, leading to decreased levels of magnesium in the body.[60] Consequently, individuals with low stomach acid may be at a higher risk of magnesium deficiency, even if they consume magnesium-rich foods or supplements. This underscores the importance of addressing issues related to stomach acid levels to ensure adequate magnesium absorption and overall health.[59]

The widespread use of proton pump inhibitors represents a significant factor contributing to low stomach acid and magnesium deficiency in today's society. Proton pump inhibitors are medications that stop the stomach from making too much acid. These medications help treat issues like ulcers, acid reflux, and conditions like Barrett's esophagus. While they can effectively alleviate symptoms associated with acid reflux and gastroesophageal reflux disease (GERD), they also suppress stomach acid secretion to unnaturally low levels.[61] This reduction in stomach acid impairs the body's ability to adequately absorb magnesium from dietary sources and supplements. Consequently, individuals taking proton pump inhibitors may be at an increased risk of magnesium deficiency. Research has highlighted the association between proton pump inhibitor use and decreased magnesium levels in the body.[60] This emphasizes the importance of monitoring magnesium status in patients on long-term therapy of proton pump inhibitors to prevent magnesium deficiency-related complications.

Kidney Disturbances

Conditions such as renal (kidney) tubular acidosis, metabolic acidosis, diabetic acidosis, prolonged diuresis, acute pancreatitis, hyperparathyroidism and primary aldosteronism can also lead to magnesium deficiency.[1, 62, 63] These conditions disrupt the magnesium balance in the body by either impairing magnesium absorption or increasing urinary excretion, contributing to magnesium deficiency over time.[63] For children with type 1 diabetes, increased urination and increased magnesium excretion due to high glucose levels and kidney tubule damage often result in intracellular magnesium deficiency, as confirmed by the intravenous magnesium tolerance test.[64] It has also been shown that patients with type 2 diabetes also tend to have lower magnesium levels compared to healthy individuals.[65]

Metabolic Acidosis

Metabolic acidosis is a condition characterized by an imbalance in the body's acid-base levels, leading to an excess of acid or a decrease in bicarbonate levels.[62, 66] This disturbance in the body's pH balance can result from various factors, including diet, kidney dysfunction, diabetes, and certain medications. Metabolic acidosis can disrupt normal physiological processes and has been linked to several health complications, including magnesium deficiency.[67]

Metabolic acidosis occurs when the body produces too much acid or when it cannot effectively remove acid through normal metabolic processes.[66] This can occur due to conditions such as kidney disease, diabetes, severe dehydration, or the ingestion of certain toxins. In metabolic acidosis, the excess acid overwhelms the body's buffering systems, leading to a decrease in blood pH.[68] As a compensatory mechanism, the body may mobilize magnesium from its stores to help neutralize the acid and restore pH balance. This increased demand for magnesium can deplete magnesium levels in the body over time, contributing to magnesium deficiency.[68] Additionally, metabolic acidosis can impair the absorption of magnesium in the gastrointestinal tract, further exacerbating magnesium deficiency.[66] It is important to address the underlying root cause of metabolic acidosis to prevent magnesium deficiency and subsequent symptoms.

Chronic Stress

In today's fast-paced society, stress has become an increasingly prevalent factor affecting individuals of all ages and backgrounds. From the demands of work and school to the challenges of personal relationships and societal pressures, stress manifests in various forms and it can impact overall well-being. It's important to recognize that stress not only affects mental and emotional health but it also has profound implications for physical health, including mineral balance within the body. Magnesium plays a crucial role in numerous physiological processes and it is intimately linked to the stress response. This is why stress can be a significant factor contributing to magnesium deficiency in the body.[69] When we are under stress, our bodies release stress hormones like cortisol, which can lead to increased magnesium excretion through the urine.[69] Furthermore, adrenaline, also known as epinephrine, is a hormone released by the adrenal glands in response to stress or danger. While adrenaline is crucial for the body's fight-or-flight response, its release can also deplete magnesium levels.[69] During periods of stress or intense physical activity, the body's demand for adrenaline increases, leading to the mobilization of magnesium from cells and tissues.[70] Magnesium plays a critical role in regulating the release and function of adrenaline, acting as a natural antagonist to counteract its effects. However, this process can result in the depletion of magnesium stores, especially when stress becomes chronic or prolonged.[70] As magnesium levels decline, the body may struggle to modulate the effects of adrenaline effectively, potentially contributing to a range of stress-related health issues.

Additionally, stress can also deplete magnesium stores because magnesium is essential for regulating stress responses and maintaining relaxation. In times of stress, the body will require more magnesium to cope with the increased demand for energy and to support the functioning of the nervous system.[69] Moreover, chronic stress can often lead to poor dietary habits, such as increased consumption of processed foods and caffeine, which are low in magnesium and can further exacerbate the deficiency of this mineral.

Caffeine and Alcohol

Caffeine and alcohol are part of everyday life for many people around the world. Caffeine, found in coffee, tea, energy drinks, and various beverages and foods, is often consumed to enhance alertness, boost energy levels, and improve cognitive function. Its stimulating effects make it a popular choice for individuals seeking a quick pick-me-up throughout the day. Conversely, alcohol, present in beer, wine, spirits, and cocktails, is commonly associated with social gatherings, celebrations, and relaxation. However, understanding their potential impact on health and their association with magnesium deficiency, is essential for maintaining overall well-being.

Substances like caffeine and alcohol are recognized for their diuretic properties. Diuretics are known to increase urine production, leading to more frequent urination. While moderate consumption may not pose significant health risks, excessive intake of alcohol and caffeine can contribute to magnesium deficiency.[71] Alcohol inhibits the release of vasopressin (also known as anti-diuretic hormone), which is responsible for water retention, thereby promoting dehydration and magnesium loss through increased urine output.[71, 72] Similarly, caffeine acts as a diuretic by blocking the action of adenosine, a hormone that regulates kidney function, resulting in enhanced urine production and some magnesium excretion.[69, 73, 74] Chronic consumption of alcohol and caffeine, especially in large quantities, can disrupt magnesium balance in the body, potentially leading to deficiency over time. Therefore, it's crucial to consume these diuretics in moderation and ensure adequate magnesium intake through diet and supplementation to maintain overall health.

Magnesium Deficient Soil and Processed Foods

Magnesium deficiency can also be attributed to depleted mineral content in soil, modern agricultural practices, and a dietary shift towards processed foods. The mineral content in soil has declined over the years due to intensive farming methods and the use of chemical fertilizers, which compromises the availability of essential nutrients like magnesium in crops.[75] Consequently, even naturally magnesium-rich foods may not offer sufficient levels of this vital mineral.[76] Moreover, processing and manufacturing techniques strip magnesium from foods, further exacerbating the deficiency.[75] Highly refined and processed foods, which dominate many diets today, tend to be low in magnesium. As a result, individuals may struggle to meet their magnesium requirements solely through dietary sources[75], especially when considering the additional depletion of magnesium by factors such as stress, absorption issues and certain medications.

Calcium and Vitamin D Supplementation

Calcium supplementation, often touted for its bone health benefits, can inadvertently lead to magnesium deficiency in the body. The relationship between calcium and magnesium is tightly regulated, and excessive calcium intake can disrupt this balance.[77] When large doses of calcium supplements are consumed without adequate magnesium intake, the body may prioritize calcium absorption over magnesium absorption, leading to magnesium depletion.[77] Furthermore, calcium and magnesium compete for absorption in the intestines, and an excess of calcium can hinder the absorption of magnesium.[78]

The widespread consumption of calcium supplements, fortified foods, and dairy products exacerbates the risk of magnesium deficiency among individuals. Many people consume more calcium than necessary through these sources, often exceeding recommended daily allowances. This creates a two-fold problem: not only does it contribute to magnesium deficiency, but it also increases the risk of calcification conditions, such as arterial calcification and kidney stones.[78] These conditions arise when excess calcium is deposited in tissues, leading to stiffness and impaired function.

Similarly, high doses of vitamin D supplementation can also contribute to magnesium deficiency. Vitamin D plays a crucial role in calcium metabolism and absorption, promoting the utilization of calcium in the body. However, excessive vitamin D levels can disrupt the delicate balance between calcium and magnesium.[79] Vitamin D enhances the absorption of calcium in the intestines, which in turn can increase the demand for magnesium to maintain proper balance.[78] As a result, prolonged high-dose vitamin D supplementation can deplete magnesium stores in the body, exacerbating the risk of magnesium deficiency.[79]

While calcium and vitamin D supplementation are often advocated for bone health, the imbalance between calcium and magnesium can have adverse effects on overall health and increase the risk of calcification conditions. Therefore, it is crucial to maintain a proper balance of these minerals through dietary sources and mindful supplementation.

Metabolic Health

Metabolic syndrome is defined by various factors including high blood pressure, blood sugar, adiposity and triglyceride levels. It is increasingly becoming a concern among the general population. A meta-analysis involving nearly 5500 patients revealed that individuals with metabolic syndrome tend to have lower magnesium levels compared to those without the syndrome.[80] In a study done in 2022, it showed that only 6.8% of U.S. adults had optimal cardiometabolic health.[81]

Overconsuming added sugars can lead to insulin resistance, which contributes to metabolic disorders like type 2 diabetes and cardiovascular disease.[82, 83] It is characterized by the cells' reduced response to insulin and it significantly contributes to magnesium deficiency by reducing the ability of magnesium to get into the cell.[84, 85] When cells resist insulin, they also struggle to absorb glucose efficiently, leading to higher blood sugar levels.[86] This imbalance triggers various physiological reactions, including increased magnesium loss through urine.[85] The depletion of magnesium caused by insulin resistance worsens the malfunction of insulin-sensitive tissues, perpetuating a cycle of metabolic problems.[86] Elevated insulin, which typically occurs after insulin resistance, also increases the urinary loss of magnesium. [87] Therefore, addressing insulin resistance through lifestyle changes and specific treatments is essential to restore magnesium levels and improve overall metabolic well-being.

Medications

Medications can also contribute to magnesium deficiency, and unfortunately, this issue is often treated with more medication. Medications can deplete magnesium by competing for intestinal absorption, increasing magnesium demand or increasing magnesium excretion.[71] Some common medications that reduce magnesium levels include birth control pills, corticosteroids, diuretics (for high blood pressure), statins (for cholesterol), insulin, and proton pump inhibitors (for acid reflux).[71] Diuretic medications, commonly prescribed to manage conditions like hypertension and edema, work by increasing urine production and promoting the excretion of water and electrolytes from the body.[88]

Since these medications are commonly prescribed, it is not surprising that magnesium deficiency is so common. Given the ever increasing number of drugs on the market and the frequency at which they are used, it is important to place greater attention on the adverse effects of drug therapy on magnesium status in order to minimize the potential health risks to individuals.

Intense Physical Exercise

Intense physical exercise, while beneficial for overall health and fitness, can also lead to depletion of magnesium levels in the body. Athletes, known for their rigorous training regimens and intense physical exertion, are therefore susceptible to magnesium deficiency. During strenuous exercise, the body undergoes various physiological changes, including increased magnesium utilization for energy production, muscle contraction, and protein synthesis.[89] Moreover, intense physical activity promotes magnesium loss through sweat, as magnesium is one of the electrolytes lost during perspiration.[89] The loss of magnesium through sweat is around 2-3 fold higher in those who are on a low sodium diet.[90] This is because magnesium is lost in sweat rather than sodium as a means to preserve sodium. This combination of increased demand and enhanced excretion can result in magnesium deficiency, especially if dietary intake or supplementation is inadequate to replenish the lost magnesium stores.

More than 42% of young athletes, including volleyball players and rowers aged 15–18 years, are deficient in magnesium, based on the oral magnesium load test.[91] The study authors believe that this test is a better indicator of magnesium deficiency compared to blood tests, especially in cases of mild deficiency. Typically, athletes lose approximately 15 mg of magnesium through sweat each day, but this amount could be higher in hot and humid conditions or during vigorous exercise.[92]

This highlights the importance of adequate magnesium intake to support optimal performance and recovery. Therefore, athletes and physically active individuals should consider monitoring their magnesium levels and ensuring sufficient dietary magnesium intake to support their training demands and overall health.

The multifaceted nature of magnesium deficiency underscores the importance of addressing its various causes to rectify deficiencies and enhance overall health. As highlighted throughout this discussion, magnesium deficiency can stem from a myriad of factors, ranging from underlying medical conditions, stress and medication use. By recognizing and addressing these contributors, individuals can take proactive steps toward restoring optimal magnesium levels and mitigating associated health risks.

Table 1 serves as a comprehensive reference, delineating both common and lesser-known causes of magnesium deficiency, providing insights for healthcare practitioners and individuals alike. Through a holistic approach that considers dietary habits, lifestyle factors, and medical history, individuals can better navigate the complexities of magnesium deficiency and pave the way for improved health outcomes.

Table 1 - Causes of Magnesium Deficiency [1, 10]

Alcohol [93]
Aldosteronism [10, 94]
Aging [95] (decreased acid in the stomach)
Antacids [95, 96] (ranitidine, famotidine, omeprazole, etc.)
Bariatric surgery [97]
Calcium (excessive intake from food or supplements)
Caffeine [98]

Cancer [99]
Celiac disease [100]
Colon removal [101]
Chronic stress [102]
Cisplatin [103-107]
Crohn's disease [108]
Cyclosporine [109-112]
Type 1 and Type 2 Diabetes [65, 113] (uncontrolled glucose levels)
Diarrhea
Diet high in fat or sugar [98, 114]
Digoxin [115]
Diuretics [116-118] (thiazide and loop diuretics)
Excessive ingestion of poorly absorbable magnesium [119] (such as magnesium oxide) leading to diarrhea and magnesium loss
Emotional and/or psychological stress [120] (overactivation of the sympathetic nervous system)
Excessive or prolonged lactation [121]
Excessive menstruation [98]
Fasting [122] (or low magnesium intake)
Foscarnet [123]
Gentamicin [124] and Tobramycin [125]
Hyperparathyroidism and hypoparathyroidism
Hyperthyroidism
Kidney diseases [126-128] (glomerulonephritis, pyelonephritis, hydronephrosis, nephrosclerosis and renal tubular acidosis)
Heart failure [129]
Hemodialysis [130]
High phosphorus in the diet [98] (soda)
Hyperinsulinemia [87] (and insulin therapy [123])
Insulin resistance [84] (intracellular magnesium depletion)
Laxatives [29]

Low salt intake [131]
Low selenium intake [98]
Gastrointestinal disorders [132] (malabsorption syndromes e.g., celiac's, nontropical sprue, bowel resection, Crohn's, ulcerative colitis, steatorrhea and prolonged diarrhea or vomiting)
Liver disease [133] (acute or chronic liver disease including cirrhosis)
Metabolic acidosis [67, 113, 134] (latent or clinical)
Pancreatitis [135-138] (acute and chronic)
Parathyroidectomy
Pentamide [123]
Peritoneal dialysis [139]
Porphyria with inappropriate secretion of antidiuretic hormone
Pregnancy
Proton pump inhibitors [140, 141]
Strenuous Exercise [142]
Tacrolimus [123]
Vitamin B6 (pyridoxine) deficiency [143, 144]
Vitamin D excess or deficiency [79, 98, 128, 145] (chronic kidney disease and liver disease can prevent the activation of vitamin D)

Potential Clinical Signs and Symptoms of Magnesium Deficiency

Recognizing the signs of magnesium deficiency is crucial for maintaining optimal health, as this mineral plays a pivotal role in numerous bodily functions. From mild symptoms to more severe manifestations, magnesium deficiency can present itself in various ways, impacting overall well-being. Understanding the spectrum of clinical signs associated with magnesium deficiency is necessary for effective management.

Magnesium deficiency can present with a variety of clinical signs and symptoms, making it a challenge sometimes to diagnose. Common indicators of magnesium deficiency include muscle cramps/twitching, spasms, and tremors, fasciculations (brief spontaneous contraction that affects a small number of muscle fibers) along with fatigue, weakness, and irritability.[1] Mental disturbances such as depression, anxiety, confusion, convulsive seizures and cognitive impairment may also occur.[63] These symptoms can often be confused with other health issues, leading to a potential misdiagnosis. Magnesium is involved in over 600 enzymatic reactions in the body, impacting various physiological processes, including muscle and nerve function, energy production, and protein synthesis.[8] Therefore, a magnesium deficiency can manifest in diverse ways. It's crucial to monitor for these signs, especially in individuals at risk of magnesium deficiency, such as those with gastrointestinal disorders, kidney disease, or certain medications that deplete the body of magnesium. Understanding these clinical manifestations can aid in timely intervention and treatment.

A common sign of magnesium deficiency in lab tests include low levels of potassium and calcium, as well as reduced magnesium in urine and/or feces. A notable and common neurological side effect with magnesium deficiency is the Trousseau sign. It involves inducing muscle spasms in the hand and forearm by occluding the brachial artery with a blood pressure cuff. When blood flow is restricted and the patient has low calcium levels this will trigger muscle spasms in the hand and forearm. A positive Trousseau's sign will make the wrist and metacarpophalangeal joints (knuckles) flex, the distal interphalangeal (DIP) and proximal interphalangeal (PIP) joints extend and the fingers adduct (brings them together).[146] The DIP joint is the one nearest the tips of the fingers. The PIP joint is the middle joint in the fingers.

A full list of potential clinical and laboratory signs of magnesium deficiency are summarized below.

Signs of Magnesium Deficiency [1, 38, 147-149]

Less severe signs[1]

- Aggression[98]
- Anxiety
- Ataxia (lack of coordination, loss of balance, trouble walking, etc.)
- Chvostek sign[63] (twitching of the facial muscles in response to tapping over the area of the facial nerve)
- Confusion

- Cramps (especially in the hands and feet)
- Disorientation
- Fasciculations ("a brief, spontaneous contraction affecting a small number of muscle fibers, often causing a flicker of movement under the skin. It can be a symptom of disease of the motor neurons"[150])
- Hyperreflexia (overactive reflex response)
- Irritability
- Muscular weakness
- Neuromuscular irritability
- Pain or hyperalgesia[151] (decreases the nociceptive threshold)
- Photosensitivity[152]
- Spasticity
- Tetany[148] (involuntary contraction of muscles)
- Tinnitus[153] (ringing in the ears)
- Tremors
- Trousseau sign
- Vertigo
- Vitamin D resistance (magnesium is needed to activate vitamin D)

Severe signs[1]

- Arrhythmias (especially Torsades de Pointes or ventricular tachycardia with a prolonged QT interval)
- Calcifications (soft tissue)
- Cataracts [154]
- Convulsions
- Coronary artery disease
- Depressed immune response [155]
- Depression [156]
- Hearing loss [98, 157]
- Heart Failure
- Hypertension

- Migraines/headaches

- Mitral valve prolapse [158]

- Osteoporosis

- Parathyroid hormone resistance and impaired parathyroid hormone release/function [159]

- Psychotic behavior

- Seizures [160] [161])

- Sudden cardiac death

- Tachycardia

Lab and EKG Signs of Magnesium Deficiency[1, 147]

- Hypomagnesemia

- Hypocalcemia

- Hypokalemia

- Prolonged QTc

- ST-segment depression[162] (in animals)

Diagnosing Magnesium Deficiency

Diagnosing subacute or chronic magnesium deficiency can be difficult because symptoms are generally non-specific. The tissues that are damaged by depletion of this mineral are those of the cardiovascular, renal, and neuromuscular systems and thus early damage is not always detectable. It is theorized that extended periods of inadequate magnesium intake might contribute to the development of chronic diseases affecting these systems.[92] In addition, there are many contributing factors and there's no one test to definitively diagnose magnesium deficiency.

Diagnosing magnesium deficiency involves a spectrum of methods, ranging from reliable yet invasive procedures to less reliable approaches. While some diagnostic techniques offer better measurements in identifying magnesium deficiency, they may require invasive procedures or specialized testing facilities. On the other hand, less reliable methods might be more accessible but may lack accuracy and precision in detecting magnesium deficiency. The choice of diagnostic method ultimately depends on various factors, including the severity of deficiency, available resources, and patient preference. It is important to acknowledge that there is not a single test that's flawless or universally perfect for diagnosing magnesium deficiency.

The more reliable methods for testing magnesium deficiency include the Thoren's intravenous magnesium load test, assessing mononuclear blood cell magnesium and muscle magnesium content through a muscle biopsy.[1] As noted earlier, while these methods are more reliable, they still come with their own limitations and challenges.

Thoren Intravenous Magnesium Load Test

Thoren proposed a method to check for magnesium deficiency using an intravenous magnesium load. If less than 70% of a dose ranging from 30 mEq to 40 mEq (approximately 365 mg to 486 mg) given to an adult over one hour is excreted in the urine over the next 16 hours, it could indicate magnesium deficiency.[163] Simply put, if you give around 400 mg of magnesium intravenously over one hour and 70% or more of that dose (280 mg or more) is not excreted in the urine within 16 hours, it suggests magnesium deficiency, even if blood magnesium levels appear normal.[38] A drawback of this test is that it is not accurate for certain patients with kidney issues where they are spilling magnesium out in their urine. These individuals may appear to have magnesium replete but are actually magnesium deficient.

Healthy individuals have been shown to retain between 2% and 8% of magnesium from an intravenous magnesium load.[44] Another study found that healthy patients, aged 18 to 66 years old, retained an average of 6.3% magnesium from such a load, with 27.5% as the upper limit for most people.[164] These findings strongly suggest that retaining over 27.5% of magnesium from an intravenous magnesium load indicates magnesium deficiency. Surprisingly, and as mentioned previously, many individuals considered healthy may actually be deficient in magnesium. For instance, in another study, young controls retained 6% magnesium, while the elderly retained 28%, indicating a significant deficiency among older adults.[165] The study's authors concluded that many healthy elderly people had a subclinical magnesium deficiency that was not picked up by standard blood tests. Magnesium deficiency in older adults has been linked to a higher risk of cardiovascular issues, osteoporosis, muscle weakness, and cognitive decline.[8]

Maintaining optimal magnesium levels is crucial for the elderly to support bone health, muscle function, heart rhythm regulation, and cognitive function.[8]

Mononuclear Blood Cell Magnesium

The Mononuclear Blood Cell Magnesium test helps diagnose magnesium deficiency by measuring the amount of magnesium in the mononuclear cells of the blood.[166] Mononuclear cells are a type of white blood cell (lymphocytes and monocytes) that can store magnesium.[166] By analyzing the magnesium content in these cells, healthcare providers can assess the body's magnesium levels more accurately than through standard blood tests alone. Low levels of magnesium in mononuclear cells indicate a whole body magnesium deficiency[167], which can help guide treatment and supplementation strategies. This test provides a more comprehensive understanding of magnesium status in the body compared to serum magnesium tests.[166]

Muscle Magnesium Content (Muscle Biopsy)

Muscle magnesium content, assessed through a muscle biopsy, involves the collection and analysis of a small sample of muscle tissue to determine the concentration of magnesium present.[168] This method is used to diagnose magnesium deficiency by measuring the actual magnesium levels within the muscle cells.

The rationale behind this approach is that magnesium plays essential roles in muscle function, including muscle contraction and relaxation.[8] Additionally, a large portion of magnesium is stored in the skeletal muscle, therefore, low levels of magnesium in muscle tissue are suggestive of systemic magnesium deficiency.[168] However, a muscle biopsy is an invasive procedure and may not be routinely performed unless there is a specific clinical indication or suspicion of magnesium deficiency that cannot be confirmed through other less invasive methods.

Less Reliable Methods of Diagnosing Magnesium Deficiency

Less reliable methods of diagnosing magnesium deficiency are also available. They are less invasive, easier to perform, and provide accessible options for healthcare providers to assess magnesium levels in patients.

Other ways to test for a magnesium deficiency: (from best to worst):[1]

- **Hair magnesium content**[169] - this can be done through a Hair Tissue Mineral Analysis (HTMA). This was shown to be an easier, cheaper and less invasive indicator of body magnesium deficiency.[170]

- **Bone magnesium** - depletion of magnesium in the coccyx may indicate magnesium deficiency.[13, 171]

- **Ratio of ionized magnesium to total magnesium** (serum or plasma[172])

This refers to the proportion of magnesium ions that are in their ionized form compared to the total amount of magnesium present in a sample or biological system. This ratio is often used to evaluate the balance between ionized and bound magnesium in the body, which can provide insights into magnesium metabolism and potential deficiencies.[172]

- **Ionized magnesium levels**[173, 174] - Whether measured in serum or erythrocytes, ionized magnesium represents the physiologically active magnesium not bound to proteins. However, this biomarker is subject to controversy and is not consistently available in clinical laboratories, making it challenging to measure reliably.

- **Lymphocyte magnesium**[175]

- **Urinary or fecal magnesium excretion**[13, 147] (low or high levels may indicate deficiency).

- **Urinary fractional magnesium excretion >4%**[176] (some studies have suggested >2% in those with normal kidney function).[177]

- **Total erythrocyte magnesium levels**[178] - It has been suggested that magnesium deficiency is indicated when erythrocyte magnesium levels fall below 1.65 mmol/L.[18]

- **Total serum magnesium levels**

It's crucial to understand that relying solely on one method (whether reliable or less reliable) to measure magnesium deficiency is not enough for an accurate diagnosis. Ideally, symptoms of magnesium deficiency will be present along with the use of more reliable tests, like intravenous or oral magnesium load, mononuclear blood cell, or muscle tests. However, symptoms may not always present. Thus, using two or more reliable measurements together can better support the diagnosis of magnesium deficiency.

Treatment of Magnesium Deficiency

Magnesium deficiency can lead to various health issues, so it's essential to address it effectively. Treatment typically involves magnesium supplementation, either through oral or intravenous administration, depending on the severity of the deficiency.[179] Oral magnesium supplements are widely available and can be taken in different forms and doses. It's essential to note that the absorption of magnesium supplements can vary, and some forms may be better tolerated than others. In severe cases or when oral supplementation is ineffective, intravenous magnesium therapy may be necessary to rapidly restore magnesium levels.[179]

In one study it was concluded that when starting magnesium replacement therapy, it's important to begin with a minimum dose of 600 mg of magnesium per day. Treatment should continue for over a month, followed by a dosage that maintains the serum magnesium level at no lower than 0.9 mmol/L.[52] They also found that using a cut-off of 0.75 mmol/L for magnesium deficiency misses half of those with a true magnesium deficiency.[52]

Improving magnesium status through diet remains a fundamental approach despite concerns about declining mineral content in our food and soils. While it's true that modern agricultural practices have led to magnesium depletion in our food, incorporating magnesium-rich foods into one's diet can still be an effective means of increasing magnesium intake.[75] Foods such as leafy greens, nuts, seeds, whole grains, and legumes are considered "high" in magnesium. However, it is important to understand that the bioavailability of magnesium in plant foods is less than animal foods (e.g., fish, shellfish, meat). Additionally, opting for organic produce whenever possible may offer slightly higher mineral content and less heavy metals and pesticides.

Addressing underlying causes of magnesium deficiency, such as dietary factors, lifestyle factors or medication use, is also essential for long-term management.

Conclusion

Subclinical magnesium deficiency is a common and often overlooked issue worldwide.[1] It's a problem that doesn't show clear symptoms, so doctors may not easily recognize it. In a time when medical costs are soaring due to extensive investments in cutting-edge technologies, it's astounding that a deficiency in one of the most inexpensive nutrients, magnesium, could underlie numerous health issues causing significant suffering and financial burdens worldwide.[98] One researcher put it rather nicely; eliminating magnesium deficiency "...may produce a higher return on investment and a higher reduction of disease and pain, in a shorter time, than any miracle drug or high-tech development."[98]

We know that even without obvious signs, subclinical magnesium deficiency can lead to serious health issues such as cardiovascular disease, brain and mood disorders, insulin resistance, metabolic syndrome, diabetes, decreased kidney function and poor bone health. We will be covering each of these in more detail in the following chapters.

A greater public health effort is needed to inform both patients and clinicians about how common and harmful a diagnosis of subclinical magnesium deficiency can be. This awareness can lead to early detection, appropriate management, and ultimately better health outcomes for individuals at risk of subclinical magnesium deficiency.

Chapter 2: Magnesium, Hard Water and Your Heart

Numerous factors can influence the risk of developing heart disease throughout one's lifetime. Besides genetic predisposition, lifestyle factors like smoking, physical inactivity, stress levels, and environmental pollution can all play significant roles. However, what you consume, both in terms of food and drink, may exert the most significant influence because they determine your intake of essential micronutrients. The mineral content of your diet and water intake largely determines your current state of health. While about 20 percent of your daily fluid intake comes from food, the remainder comes from what you drink. In addition, recommendations regarding water consumption can vary widely. Let's face it, if you prefer hydrating foods like watermelons and salads, which have high water content, you will likely feel less thirsty compared to a meal composed of a burger and fries. Yet, here's a question for you; how often have you considered the quality of the water you drink and use for cooking daily? Furthermore, do you have any concerns about your local water quality?

Almost 60 years ago, researchers Morris, Crawford, and Heady were among the first to unveil an association between water quality, specifically the hardness of local water sources, and cardiovascular related deaths. Their crucial research, which was published in 1961, established a direct connection between human health and the mineral content of local water sources.[180] Margaret Crawford, the lead researcher, was a pioneer in the field of cardiovascular epidemiology, and spearheaded groundbreaking research in 1968 with her colleagues. Together, they had uncovered a strong association between mortality rates related to cardiovascular diseases and the softness of water supplies. Notably, their studies highlighted an elevated risk of cardiovascular disease in areas with low calcium water sources.[181, 182]

In 1981, Masironi and Shaper provided further evidence of this association, referencing 11 publications from different parts of the world. They demonstrated that populations consuming higher mineral content waters experienced reduced rates of heart attacks and deaths from various cardiovascular conditions, including arteriosclerosis, coronary heart disease, and hypertensive heart disease.[182] The U.S. Environmental Protection

Agency conducted a similar investigation across 35 separate geographic regions in the United States and noted that water hardness and calcium levels correlated with lower mortality rates from cardiovascular diseases.[183] Essentially, the message is clear; the higher the mineral content in drinking water, the lower the rate of death from cardiovascular disease.

First, we need to clarify what contributes to the hardness of water. Monovalent cations (monovalent meaning one charge) like sodium (Na+), potassium (K+), and lithium (Li+) do not contribute to water hardness because they have a valency, or bonding ability, of one. These atoms can only form one chemical bond because they can either lose or gain only one electron to become stable. On the other hand, divalent cations (divalent meaning two charges) like calcium (Ca^{2+}) or magnesium (Mg^{2+}) do contribute to water hardness because they have a valency of two. They can form two chemical bonds because they can either lose or gain two electrons to get a stable electron configuration.[184]

Here's a simple definition for the difference between soft and hard water. You can rate your local water supply using the following:[182]

- **Soft water:** Calcium carbonate concentration below 75 mg/L

- **Hard water**: Calcium carbonate concentration > 100 mg/L

- **Very hard water**: Calcium carbonate concentration > 200 mg/L

It is important to understand that while drinking waters may have a similar total level of hardness, their concentrations of calcium and magnesium can vary significantly.[182] We will explore this topic further in the upcoming sections of this chapter.

These days, soft water is the primary choice for many of us. Its popularity stems from its practicality and straightforward benefits, explaining why softer waters have gained widespread acceptance in industrialized societies. Soft water reduces the need for soap, whether it is for personal hygiene, laundry or when washing dishes. It also minimizes the buildup of scale in pipes and leaves fewer stains on pots, pans, and enamel sinks. However, there's a downside to soft water. It can corrode and dissolve some of the metals found in water distribution pipes over time, thereby releasing substances like copper, zinc, and cadmium into the water supply.[182] Researchers, Masironi and Shaper, have noted that soft water could contain trace amounts of toxic elements from pipes or soil, while hard water might offer protection due to its calcium and magnesium content, along with beneficial trace elements.[182] An interesting historical example comes from Cornish mineworkers who found relief from lead-induced gout when they moved to a region that naturally provided harder spring water. They effectively cleansed and detoxified by switching from tainted soft water to calcium-rich hard water. Today, in regions with hard water, calcium from the water supply can actually help prevent the leaching of toxins from lead piping.

Other factors may also be involved in the effects of water hardness. Some experts suggest that the negative impact of soft water could be partly due to increased cadmium levels (cadmium is a toxic heavy metal), while others argue that the protective benefits of hard water come from higher levels of minerals like chromium, iodine, and lithium.[182] Additionally, many researchers highlight the absence of magnesium in the soft water supply as a key factor for the association with worse health outcomes.

The Food Mineral Hypothesis vs. The Water Mineral Hypothesis

It has long been believed that our food contains enough minerals to support our overall well-being. However, historically, water has also been recognized as a valuable mineral source for both humans and animals, that is until the softening of water became common. Consuming water that is rich in minerals offers an effective means to fulfill your nutritional needs while optimizing nutrient intake without excessive calorie consumption. We can think of high-mineral water as nature's original multivitamin, but we need to make sure to get a daily source of those waters from trustworthy sources.

We are not just referring to drinking water here. To maximize the benefits of water that is rich in minerals, it should also be used in cooking and the preparation of foods. When we boil pasta, rice, and vegetables in such water it increases their mineral content, as food absorbs water during cooking. It is worth noting that dry pasta nearly doubles in weight when boiled, while white rice can even triple its weight. Since the chemical makeup of your cooking water impacts the food you eat, using water that is lacking in minerals (passing through a water softener) can result in cooked food that has less minerals. Conversely, food will gain minerals when cooked in hard water.[182] The bottom line? **It is beneficial to cook your food in hard water in addition to drinking hard water.**

Mineral-to-Toxic Heavy Metal Ratios Matter More Than Absolute Values

Crawford highlights the importance of higher calcium levels in water for two key reasons. Firstly, they are believed to inhibit the absorption of harmful elements from pipes and soil, as hard water is less corrosive than soft water. This means that with hard waters, especially those with elevated calcium levels, there is less leaching of metals like lead and cadmium from water pipes, offering a protective effect. Secondly, the body's absorption of toxic metals such as lead and cadmium is inversely linked to the concentration of calcium. Therefore, high-calcium water may offer a dual protective effect, reducing the presence of toxic heavy metals and limiting their absorption into the body.[182] In simple terms, although the calcium-rich 'hard' water may cause some inconvenience by causing scaling in water pipes and kitchen appliances such as coffee makers, it is precisely this calcium lining that prevents any leaching, providing us that double protection.

Minerals Present in Water are Easier Absorbed by the Body Compared to Those Obtained From Food and Supplements.

Many of us obtain calcium from our diets. According to the U.S. National Institutes of Health a significant portion of Americans (43%) also take a regular supplement which includes calcium.[185] However, even if your diet lacks calcium, your drinking water might provide a substantial amount of this mineral. Research by Crawford reveals that in the UK, areas with hard water can offer up to 2 grams more calcium daily compared to soft-water areas, which represents a significant factor. While not all ingested calcium is absorbed by the body, it is estimated that less than 30% from food sources is typically absorbed. Considering various absorption factors, the importance of water emerges as a vital calcium source. This may be greater than most of us appreciate.[182] Notably, the body struggles to process large calcium doses at once, highlighting the steady supply from hard water as preferable over sporadic calcium pill consumption.[186] Bottom line?

Minerals from water are more readily absorbed by the body compared to those from food and supplements.

The Magnesium Present in Mineral Waters Could be Key to Promoting Optimal Heart Health.

When you think of "hard water," you likely envision the tough scaled residue calcium leaves on pipes and appliances, but there's a second mineral involved and that is magnesium. Although calcium usually plays a bigger role, water with low calcium but high magnesium content falls under the category of hard water. The impact of getting more magnesium for our health is profound; while the connection between calcium and heart health is mostly down to correlation, the hypothesis strongly supports magnesium as a heart-healthy mineral. This is supported by findings indicating that individuals who passed away due to ischemic heart disease exhibited a 24% lower magnesium concentration in the myocardium compared to those who died from accidents. In other words, people who die from heart disease have less magnesium in their heart. Furthermore, men living in regions with soft water, who pass away from accidents, exhibit lower levels of magnesium compared to those residing in hard-water areas. To clarify, the more magnesium you consume in your water the greater magnesium in your body. Animal and laboratory experiments have demonstrated the biological plausibility of this factor. However, as Masironi noted in 1981, *"It is difficult to judge whether the apparently lower magnesium content of a damaged heart is a result or a cause of that damage."[182]* It appears that magnesium deficiency could potentially be damaging to those hearts that are already compromised, while higher levels might offer protection. This notion is underscored by the following observation: "*High rates of coronary heart disease in Ohio were observed in regions with less than 15 mg of magnesium per liter in the drinking water, whereas areas with 36 mg/liter exhibited low Coronary Heart Disease rates. Similar results were reported by other researchers."[182]*

While calcium levels can be abundant, particularly in modern processed foods that are often calcium-fortified, the magnesium content tends to be much lower. The recommended daily intake levels of magnesium are rarely achieved. Consuming a typical Western diet (includes most Americans), makes it challenging for individuals to reach the recommended daily magnesium intake of 310-420 mg. While this may not always lead to an apparent magnesium deficiency, it remains a concern for many individuals. Once more, this underscores the crucial role that drinking and cooking with hard water can play. It is important to mention again that even if your water is labeled as hard, it does not guarantee that there is sufficient magnesium content. However, it is worth investigating to confirm. You can also buy water that contains magnesium (such as San Pellegrino, Gerolsteiner or Magnesia) or take magnesium supplements.

Masironi also references research from Canada that indicates that areas with high magnesium content in the water can supply up to 20% of an individual's daily magnesium intake.[182] If you reside in a region where the drinking water contains 50 mg of magnesium per liter, then consuming three liters of that water per day would give you an extra 150 mg of magnesium per day compared to someone consuming water with no magnesium in it. In contrast, European drinking water systems typically contain low magnesium levels, averaging around 12 mg/liter, contributing only about 10% to the average daily intake. In 1976, researchers Zoetman & Brinkmann noted the widespread consumption of bottled mineral water in Europe may elevate magnesium intake by up to 40% for some individuals.[182] This observation was made long before consuming bottled water became a regular part of US drinking habits, a trend that was nearly unheard of in 1976 but is now widely accepted.

The Human Body Requires a Significant Quantity of Water on a Daily Basis

As humans, we typically consume about two to three liters of water daily, especially in hotter climates. Our goal is not necessarily to urge you to drink more or more often, but rather to encourage you to maximize the benefits of your daily hydration routine. Simply quenching your natural thirst offers a valuable opportunity to absorb important and essential minerals. What an opportunity this is. On average, tap water is reported to account for approximately 60% of your body's daily fluid intake.[182]

Many of us do not consider the quality of the water we drink daily, as long as it is deemed safe. Tap water is widely accessible and free in most regions, so we drink and cook with it without much thought. However, our health may be impacted by what is in that tap water, or more commonly, by what it is lacking. The overall long-term consequences may stem from a reduced intake of vital minerals, but also an unwanted intake of heavy metals. By consuming water lacking in minerals, we inadvertently heighten the absorption and toxicity of heavy metals like aluminum, cadmium, lead, mercury, and arsenic, as well as increasing the risk of certain diseases. Notably, the higher calcium content in hard water can serve as a protective shield against the absorption of lead and cadmium.[182]

Obtaining accurate national figures proved challenging, but a 2004 household survey in Phoenix, Arizona, revealed that a quarter of households utilized water softening equipment for their daily water supply[187]; a relatively new trend at the time. Reflecting on human history, we traditionally did not consume artificially "softened" water, even when it became available through piped systems. Instead, we used to drink the naturally occurring hard water, which was richer in beneficial minerals, that nature provided quite naturally for us. The accessibility of such water is also changing. As modern agricultural practices have expanded, our soil and the water running through it have experienced a steady decline in mineral content. Consequently, the tap water we currently rely on tends to possess lower levels of the healthiest minerals than in the past. While harder water may lead to visible scaling in household kettles and pipes, its mineral-rich composition appears to specifically contribute to reduced rates of heart disease.

Referring again to Masironi's comprehensive review: *"Because of the amount taken in, as well as of the free, ionic easily absorbable form in which the chemical elements are present, water is a source of trace and major elements in human nutrition that cannot be disregarded."[182]*

Harder tap waters can provide more than 10% of the human daily requirement for elements like Lithium, Fluorine, Calcium, Copper, Magnesium, Iron, and Zinc.[182] While 10% might seem insignificant, consider this: If our food contained an abundance of minerals, one might question the significance of water's impact. However, the mineral content in our increasingly processed food supply chain has been declining over the years, prompting us to reconsider water's importance in our mineral intake. Some individuals may encounter subtle mineral deficiencies, and the extra 10% from harder water might represent the crucial distinction between life-long suboptimal health levels and optimal well-being.

Bottom Line: **Considering the heightened risk of marginal nutritional deficiencies stemming from refined foods, inadequate diets, and chronic diseases, consuming water that is rich in minerals could be the pivotal factor between enjoying optimal health and longevity or facing illness.**

A Geographical Benefit? Tap Water Sourced From the Western United States and Southern Europe Could Offer Enhanced Health Advantages.

While calcium and magnesium levels predominantly determine water hardness, a myriad of other minerals are often present as well. After conducting initial fieldwork in the early 1970s, Roberto Masironi and his colleagues went on to study the association between geographical locations and water hardness, exploring its potential link with cardiovascular disease (CVD). To the north of Europe, extensive and ancient geological formations underlie surface rocks and topsoil, resulting in naturally soft underground water flows that are low in minerals. However, further South the water becomes more hard. A comparable feature is also evident in North America, running in an East-West direction (West typically having harder water than cities in the East). In both continents, the association with cardiovascular disease (CVD) aligns with the softness of the water. The team concluded that the geographical location relative to the local geological formations consistently demonstrated comparable patterns regarding water hardness and cardiovascular disease.[182] Thus, your fate, at least to some degree, is influenced by the inherent composition of the bedrock upon which your community where you live was established.

In the USA, it's ironic to note the increasing use of water softeners, which inadvertently alters the positive heart-friendly attributes of hard water. While it makes practical sense to minimize build up of deposits in appliances and pipes, the impact on our cardiovascular health appears to tell a different story.

"...in hard water areas of the US it is estimated that 60-70% of residences use water softeners."[182] In fact, a study revealed that half of the residents in areas with naturally hard water opted for softened or bottled water of their own choice (a figure likely higher in today's context).

Is it time to reassess your preference for soft tap water? There are compelling cumulative advantages to sticking with hard water (or mineral waters) for both drinking and cooking, but there is another noteworthy benefit to consider. Beyond the numerous correlations with heart health, areas consuming soft water also exhibit higher rates of bladder or urinary tract stone formation.[182] Furthermore, in animals, more atherosclerosis (which is a build up of plaque in the arteries) occurs when given distilled water instead of hard water.[188] Could it be that soft water poses greater harm than the widely believed notion that fatty foods clog arteries?

What Underlies the Theory Linking Water Hardness to Cardiovascular Disease?

It is time to examine what is happening inside your home's water pipes. While a water softener prevents the buildup of limescale in pipes, predominantly composed of calcium carbonate, it is worth noting that soft water flowing through household pipes can also have an impact on those pipes. The slight acidity of soft water, attributed to its carbon dioxide content, gradually lends it a corrosive quality. Over time, the water develops a cumulative corrosive nature, potentially leading to the stripping of harmful elements (lead, cadmium etc.) from the piping. The extent of this process depends on the composition of the piping material. Gradually, this process leads to adverse effects on your personal cardiovascular health, offering a biologically plausible mechanism for the association between soft water supplies and cardiovascular disease. On the other hand, harder water supplies which contain calcium as well as other beneficial minerals like magnesium, are crucial for heart health and overall well-being.[182]

Little has changed since researchers in 1975 reached the conclusion: *"According to a WHO expert group, evidence from many properly designed epidemiological studies undertaken by independent investigators shows that hardness of drinking water (and particularly the calcium content) in Canada, the UK, and the US is inversely associated with cardiovascular mortality, and with adult mortality in general...This was also the conclusion of an international group of experts who met in 1975 under the auspices of the Commission of the European Communities."[182]*

The extensive work conducted by R. Masironi from the Cardiovascular Disease Unit of the World Health Organization (WHO) in Geneva, alongside A.G. Shaper from the Royal Free Hospital School of Medicine in London, represented the most comprehensive piece of research on the topic, and it remains relevant today. A team of researchers in Ontario analyzed data from various countries. They found that differences in water hardness, particularly the calcium and magnesium content of the water, were linked to approximately 10% of the variability in chronic heart disease (CHD). In regions with soft water in the US, there was a 15% higher rate of cardiovascular mortality compared to areas with hard water. The National Academy of Sciences of the US stated that "...*the body of evidence is sufficiently compelling to treat the "water story" as plausible, particularly when the number of potentially preventable deaths from cardiovascular diseases is considered."[182]* During that period in the United States, cardiovascular diseases made up over half of the roughly two million annual deaths. According to the WHO report, improving access to better quality drinking water could potentially decrease yearly cardiovascular disease mortality rates by up to 15%. However, typical of associative research, they were not prescriptive with offering specific solutions. The researchers recognized the need for more definitive information to determine the exact remedial water treatment measures that should be considered.[182]

The Crucial Importance of Magnesium

When you observe the limescale buildup in your water pipes, kettle, or coffee machine, it typically consists of calcium carbonate. However, it's the magnesium content in this buildup that could have the greatest impact on your heart health; and surprisingly, your taste buds as well. Even with Starbucks maintaining consistency in the quality and degree of their coffee bean roast across all their locations, the water's hardness could affect the taste more than you might anticipate. Hence, this is why the same coffee brand may taste different in Tampa, Florida, with its hard water ranging from 140 to 300 parts per million (note that this is very hard), compared to Portland, Oregon, known for its exceptionally soft water with typically 3 to 8 parts per million of dissolved minerals.[189] So the question is; which coffee tastes better and why?

Christopher Hendon, a chemist at the University of Bath in England, uncovered the pivotal role of water composition in extracting sugars, starches, bases, and acids from a specific coffee roast. Contrary to popular belief that hard water detracts from coffee quality, his collaboration with a local coffee shop revealed that taste was less influenced by soft or hard water and more by the specific type of hardness. According to Hendon, elevated levels of magnesium ions enhance coffee extraction and improve the taste, while excessive bicarbonate levels are detrimental.[190] His findings revealed that sodium rich waters that are produced by water softeners did not enhance taste, but magnesium-rich water proved to be superior. This research not only yielded valuable insights but also led to competitive success. Transitioning from theory to action, during the 2014 global barista championships in Rome, Maxwell Colonna-Dashwood, his barista partner, secured fifth place overall among more than 50 competitors, employing their specially chosen water.[191] If you want to know more about the impact of water on coffee, they co-authored a book titled, "Water for Coffee."

The reason you may opt for bottled water with elevated magnesium levels in your coffee maker might be primarily aimed at enhancing taste. However, the significant benefit could extend to your heart health. The Chipperfields, a collaborative husband and wife team from the biochemistry and chemistry departments at the University of Hull in England, have underscored magnesium's crucial role in heart muscle contraction and oxidative phosphorylation (energy production) in heart mitochondria. While it may seem complex, this concept is important because oxidative phosphorylation is the mechanism through which adenosine triphosphate (ATP) is formed; an essential molecule often considered as the energy currency of life. ATP serves as the high-energy compound storing the necessary energy for virtually all bodily functions, and it has been proposed that a magnesium-ATP complex serves as the true substrate for ATP-related reactions.[192]

Research has demonstrated a rapid depletion of magnesium from the heart when subjected to oxygen deprivation in controlled experiments, suggesting that a prolonged lack of blood flow to the heart (angina episodes) could deplete magnesium levels in the heart. Animal studies further reveal that a magnesium-deficient diet increases the likelihood of myocardial fiber necrosis (death of fibers in the heart); however, the administration of magnesium salts can reverse numerous associated changes. [193-196] Strong evidence suggests that administering magnesium salts beforehand can shield the heart from various alterations induced by oxygen deprivation. This provides additional support for a magnesium-rich diet in averting the detrimental effects of acute ischemic incidents like heart attacks.

There's a theory suggesting that the elevated prevalence of heart disease in Scotland, in contrast to England, may be linked to the twenty-fold greater magnesium content found in English beer compared to Scottish Whisky. However, let's leave that tale for another time!

The Relationship Between Water Hardness and Magnesium in the Heart Muscle

In general terms, it appears that lower magnesium levels in drinking water correlate with lower magnesium levels in the heart. This could potentially account for the higher occurrence of sudden cardiac deaths in regions with low magnesium content in their drinking water. A study conducted in Ontario supports this notion, where an analysis of heart muscle samples from individuals who passed away after accidents in regions with soft water revealed markedly lower concentrations of magnesium. Interestingly, when compared to individuals residing in hard water regions, those from soft water areas exhibited a lower magnesium/potassium ratio in their hearts.[182] The authors concluded that, *"Western diets are probably often low in magnesium, so that the magnesium in hard drinking water may help to protect its consumers from ischemic heart disease."* [182] While the study was not extensive, it encompassed 64 Canadian males who died from accidents and were considered representative of the general population when compared to those who succumbed to "natural causes." Among them, 20 were from three different hard-water areas, while 44 resided in five soft-water areas. The average magnesium concentrations in the wet heart tissue of individuals from hard and soft water regions were 222.3 ug/gram and 206.7 ug/gram, respectively, with a statistically significant difference observed. Another interpretation of these findings implies that while the presence of heart disease itself might contribute to decreased magnesium levels in the heart, consuming soft water, which typically contains less magnesium, also appears to correlate with reduced magnesium content.[197]

It's noteworthy that magnesium ranks as the fourth most abundant mineral in the human body, following calcium, sodium, and potassium. Among the 25 grams of magnesium found in an average 70-kilogram human (155 pounds), over half resides in the bones, a quarter in the muscle tissue, and the remainder is dispersed among soft tissue and blood.[198] As we have mentioned, a deficiency in magnesium is of significant concern. It not only impacts heart health but numerous other health conditions. Magnesium plays a vital role in efficient biochemical functioning of many metabolic pathways in the body.

The human body operates through a complex web of interdependent factors to sustain balance and well-being, and while magnesium is crucial, it's not the sole factor to consider in your water supply. Alongside the necessity for adequate calcium levels, it's important to recognize the role of sodium as well. Examining 4,200 adults across 35 geographic regions in the United States, researchers analyzed the tap water quality at each participant's residence. While the anticipated negative correlations were observed between hardness, calcium, and mortality rates for various cardiovascular diseases, they unexpectedly found that elevated sodium levels were also negatively associated with cardiovascular mortality rates among both men and women. As observed previously with magnesium, increased sodium levels in residents' tap water were also implicated in reducing the rates of mortality from cardiovascular, kidney, and ischemic heart diseases.

Undoubtedly, individual exposure to drinking water significantly impacts cardiovascular health. In the upcoming chapter, we will dive deeper into the pivotal role of magnesium as a vital mineral for overall cardiovascular health. In the meantime, if you have not already, consider reaching out to your local water authority or supplier to gain insight into the mineral composition of your daily water intake. Additionally, consider drinking more mineral waters (San Pellegrino, Gerolsteiner, Magnesia) over tap water. Discovering the specific mineral content in your daily intake of water, tea, coffee, boiled vegetables, and dry goods can provide valuable insights. It could be an enlightening experience for you, your family and your health.

Chapter 3: Magnesium and Cardiovascular Disease

Cardiovascular disease stands as a leading cause of morbidity and mortality globally, encompassing a spectrum of conditions affecting the heart and blood vessels. According to the World Health Organization, an estimated 17.9 million deaths occur annually due to cardiovascular disease, representing approximately 31% of all global deaths. These conditions include coronary artery disease, myocardial infarction (heart attack), stroke, heart failure, and peripheral arterial disease, among others.[199] Cardiovascular disease manifests through various mechanisms, often arising from a culmination of risk factors such as high blood pressure, elevated triglycerides, high insulin, poor blood sugar regulation, smoking, physical inactivity, obesity, and poor diet, among others. These risk factors can contribute to the development and progression of atherosclerosis, a condition that is characterized by the buildup of plaque within arterial walls, leading to narrowed and hardened arteries, thereby compromising blood flow to vital organs such as the heart and brain.[199]

The impact of cardiovascular disease extends far beyond mortality rates, profoundly affecting individual health and well-being while imposing substantial economic burdens on healthcare systems worldwide. Individuals affected by cardiovascular disease often experience a diminished quality of life due to symptoms such as chest pain, shortness of breath, fatigue, and limitations in physical activity.[199] Moreover, cardiovascular disease complications, including heart attacks and strokes, can result in long-term disability, necessitating costly medical interventions and rehabilitation efforts. Consequently, the prevention and management of cardiovascular disease remains imperative with public health priorities aimed at reducing both the incidence and burden of cardiovascular-related morbidity and mortality.[200]

Magnesium is an essential mineral with diverse physiological functions. It serves as a cofactor in over 600 enzymatic reactions, such as those responsible for regulating blood pressure, blood sugar control, and lipid peroxidation.[2] In addition, magnesium contributes significantly to the proper functioning of the heart and blood vessels. Therefore, it plays a critical role in supporting the cardiovascular system.[201]

In industrialized Western countries, insufficient magnesium intake often results in a higher occurrence of magnesium deficiency, which subsequently increases the likelihood of cardiovascular events and cardiovascular mortality.[202] As we have mentioned in chapter one, magnesium deficiency is a common and often under-recognized problem throughout the world. Magnesium deficiency has been implicated in the pathogenesis of various cardiovascular disorders. Research suggests that inadequate magnesium levels may contribute to endothelial dysfunction, arterial stiffness, and dysregulated cardiac rhythm, predisposing individuals to hypertension, atherosclerosis, and arrhythmias.[202, 203] Furthermore, magnesium deficiency has been associated with insulin resistance, inflammation, and oxidative stress, all of which are implicated in the development and progression of cardiovascular disease.[203, 204]

Epidemiology

Despite magnesium's crucial role in maintaining the proper functioning of the cardiovascular system, research indicates that dietary magnesium intake is frequently insufficient in the USA, a trend mirrored in North European countries. Multiple factors are believed to contribute to this trend, including the depletion of magnesium during food processing, the relatively low bioavailability of magnesium from vegetarian diets, metabolic changes associated with pregnancy, medications for osteoporosis, alcoholism, stress, and variations in the magnesium content of water.[17] The precise human dietary requirement for essential minerals like magnesium remains uncertain. Earlier balance studies suggested daily recommended magnesium intakes ranging from 300 to 354 mg/day for American women and 420 to 483 mg/day for American men.[205] However, other research indicates that around 180 mg of magnesium per day might suffice to maintain a positive magnesium balance.[28] However, being in a positive balance does not mean an optimal intake. Actual intakes among American women and men hover around 228 mg/day and 331 mg/day, respectively.[205] This is around 200-300 mg lower than what an optimal intake of magnesium should be (425-600 mg per day).[7, 9]

As mentioned in Chapter 2, there is also an interesting association between cardiovascular disease and the hardness of drinking water, primarily due to variations in magnesium content. In addition, changes in water hardness, and a transition to soft water, associate with increased rates of death from cardiovascular diseases, including heart attacks and strokes.[206]

Biochemical Interactions of Magnesium in Cardiovascular Diseases

Examining the biochemical interactions of magnesium in cardiovascular diseases offers crucial insights for both understanding and addressing heart-related issues. Due to magnesium playing such a pivotal role in maintaining heart health, it is imperative to comprehend its intricate functions within the cardiovascular system to improve prevention and treatment strategies.

Recent studies on hospitalized patients revealed that 42% were found to have hypomagnesemia (low magnesium levels).[207] However, physicians only requested magnesium testing for 7% of these patients.[207] Additionally, in a study conducted among patients in the intensive cardiac care unit, 53% exhibited mononuclear cell magnesium content below the lowest normal control.[208]

As we have mentioned, in clinical practice, serum magnesium is typically what is assessed, even though less than 1% of magnesium resides extracellularly. As a result, serum magnesium may not consistently indicate the total body magnesium stores accurately. It is known that serum magnesium levels can appear normal despite a depletion of total body magnesium content.[208] In experimental settings, determining total body magnesium stores can be estimated by measuring retention of an oral or intravenous magnesium load. However, this measurement method is complex and requires a 24-hour urine collection. In numerous instances, intracellular levels of magnesium offer a more reliable gauge for total body magnesium content compared to serum magnesium levels, with blood mononuclear cell magnesium testing being the most precise.[1] Additionally, mononuclear magnesium content demonstrates a stronger correlation with cardiac magnesium status.[209, 210]

Magnesium exerts various effects on the pathogenesis of cardiovascular diseases at biochemical and cellular levels. Initially, magnesium activates adenosine triphosphatase (ATPase), critical for cell membrane function and serving as the energy source for the Na^+–K^+ (sodium potassium) pump.[211] Studies in rats have demonstrated that magnesium deficiency reduces the Na^+–K^+ pump activity, resulting in elevated intracellular sodium levels, thus disrupting the membrane potential.[212] In their examination of sodium kinetics and membrane potential in the aorta of magnesium-deficient rats, researchers demonstrated that magnesium deficiency led to a less polarized membrane potential due to intracellular sodium accumulation, indicating potential inhibition of the Na^+–K^+ pump.[213] This alteration in membrane potential has been proposed as a potential mechanism for causing arrhythmias.

Magnesium serves as a critical cofactor essential for the proper functioning of enzymes within the mitochondria of the heart. Also, magnesium acts as a protective factor against potassium loss in the cell. Many times, low potassium in the blood is actually due to a magnesium deficiency. Insufficient intracellular magnesium levels can also result in heightened levels of intracellular sodium and calcium, contributing to conditions such as arterial vasospasm, elevated catecholamine release, increased fatty acids and lipids, as well as intravascular hypercoagulability.[211, 214]

Furthermore, magnesium deficiency has been implicated in playing a role in inflammation, as evidenced by studies conducted in rats. This research has demonstrated that as magnesium deficiency progresses, there is a notable increase in serum levels of inflammatory cytokines such as interleukin-1, interleukin-6, and tumor necrosis factor after three weeks on a magnesium-deficient diet.[215] Additionally, magnesium deficiency increases the susceptibility of all cells to oxidative stress, predisposing individuals to proatherogenic changes in lipids, endothelial dysfunction, thrombosis and hypertension.[216] All of these contribute to the pathogenesis of metabolic syndrome and cardiovascular diseases.[217]

In the upcoming sections, we will explore the different cardiovascular disorders and how magnesium, or not having enough of it, affects each one. By acknowledging these connections, we can uncover essential knowledge about maintaining heart health and appreciate the significant role magnesium plays in this process.

Hypertension

Hypertension, commonly referred to as high blood pressure, is characterized by persistently elevated pressure within the blood vessels. Blood, propelled by the heart, circulates throughout the body via these vessels. With each heartbeat, the heart pumps blood into these vessels, generating blood pressure—a measure of the force exerted by the blood against the arterial walls. Elevated blood pressure places greater strain on the heart, necessitating increased pumping effort.[218]

This medical condition poses significant health risks, including an increased risk of heart, brain, kidney, and other diseases. It stands as a leading cause of premature mortality globally, affecting over a billion individuals, with approximately 1 in 4 men and 1 in 5 women afflicted.[218]

Blood pressure is typically expressed as two numbers. The first number, known as systolic pressure, reflects the force in the blood vessels when the heart contracts or beats. Conversely, the second number, called diastolic pressure, indicates the pressure in the blood vessels when the heart rests between beats. A diagnosis of hypertension is established when, on two separate occasions, the systolic blood pressure readings are equal to or greater than 140 mmHg and/or the diastolic blood pressure readings are equal to or greater than 90 mmHg.[219]

Hypertension is a complex and multifaceted disorder with a diverse range of contributing factors. Both clinical observations and experimental research have suggested that magnesium deficiency plays a role in the pathogenesis of hypertension, particularly through an increased constriction of arterial smooth muscle. Magnesium predominantly resides at the inner surface of cell membranes. As a result, it influences the ability of cell membranes to allow the passage of sodium and calcium ions.[220] As previously mentioned magnesium activates the Na^+–K^+–ATPase pump, a critical mechanism responsible for maintaining the balance of sodium and potassium ions by facilitating the movement of potassium into the cells and sodium out of the cells. A deficiency in magnesium can result in leaky arterial and arteriolar membranes causing edema or swelling. This also contributes to a decrease in potassium levels (both in the blood and the cell) and an increase in calcium and sodium in cardiac and smooth muscle cells. Elevated intracellular calcium levels can contribute to hypertension, vasospasms, and arterial calcifications.[221]

Numerous observational and experimental studies have supported the significance of magnesium depletion in the development of hypertension. Studies conducted on magnesium-deficient rats have demonstrated the onset of hypertension.[222] Similarly, human studies have echoed these findings. For instance, a study by Shibutani et al. examined 380 Japanese junior high school students and revealed that red blood cell magnesium levels were lower in boys with a family history of hypertension compared to those without a family history of hypertension. Additionally, those with a family history of hypertension had higher blood pressure if they had lower serum and red blood magnesium compared to those with higher magnesium levels.[223] These results suggest that magnesium deficiency may contribute, at least partially, to elevated blood pressure in students with a familial predisposition to hypertension. The study also suggests that a genetic predisposition to hypertension may be closely associated with magnesium deficiency.[223]

Reduced magnesium levels can impair the function of endothelial cells (cells that line the inside of our arteries), potentially heightening the risk of thrombosis (blood clot formation) and atherosclerosis (a buildup of plaque in the arteries).[224] Additionally, magnesium deficiency can induce a proatherogenic, dysfunctional state in endothelial cells, which is a pre-requisite to plaque building up in the arteries.[225] In other words, magnesium deficiency sets the stage for heart disease. Low magnesium levels may also hinder the release of nitric oxide from the coronary endothelium, whereas magnesium therapy has been shown to improve endothelium-dependent vasodilation in individuals with coronary artery disease.[226] Given that nitric oxide serves dual roles as both a vasodilator and an inhibitor of platelet aggregation, magnesium supplementation emerges as a promising therapeutic approach for managing hypertension and coronary artery disease. Notably, magnesium therapy has the potential to enhance prostacyclin release from the vascular wall, which is important for inhibiting blood clotting.[227]

Many individuals diagnosed with hypertension or heart failure undergo treatment involving thiazide and loop diuretics, medications that lead to magnesium depletion in the body.[228] Administering oral magnesium supplementation to hypertensive patients on long-term thiazide diuretics has been shown to markedly lower blood pressure.[228] In fact, the elevated intracellular calcium levels resulting from magnesium deficiency may contribute to both insulin resistance and hypertension.[229] A meta-analysis of

59

randomized, double-blind, placebo-controlled trials involving normotensive and hypertensive adults revealed that daily magnesium supplementation of 368 mg over a median duration of three months significantly reduces systolic blood pressure by 2.00 mmHg and diastolic blood pressure by 1.78 mmHg.[230]

The impact of magnesium supplementation on patients using diuretics has been explored in various trials. Hattori et al. investigated 20 individuals with essential hypertension undergoing long-term thiazide diuretic therapy, alongside 21 untreated patients of similar age. The group receiving diuretics was supplemented with magnesium oxide (600 mg/day) for a duration of 4 weeks. Substantial reductions in intra-erythrocyte sodium levels and mean blood pressure, coupled with increased red cell magnesium content, were observed in the diuretic group receiving magnesium supplementation.[231] The effect of magnesium on lowering blood pressure was more pronounced in the subset of nine patients who showed little response to diuretic therapy.[231] A comprehensive meta-analysis pooling data from seven studies involving 135 hypertensive patients on antihypertensive medications, with an initial average blood pressure exceeding 155 mmHg, demonstrated that magnesium supplementation led to a reduction in blood pressure by -18.7/10.9 mmHg.[232] Another meta-analysis comprising 22 trials, with an average magnesium dose of 410 mg, revealed a significant decrease in both systolic (3-4 mm Hg) and diastolic (2-3 mm Hg) blood pressure. The reduction in blood pressure was more pronounced with magnesium doses exceeding 370 mg/day.[233]

Magnesium supplementation can offer a valuable therapeutic approach in managing hypertension, particularly in individuals undergoing diuretic therapy. By addressing magnesium deficiency and restoring optimal levels, it is possible to mitigate the risk of hypertension and its associated complications. Therefore, ensuring adequate magnesium intake may prove to be a beneficial and effective measure in the prevention and management of hypertension.

Atherosclerosis and Calcifications

According to the World Health Organization, atherosclerosis stands as the primary contributor to mortality, driving a range of cardiovascular and vascular ailments such as heart attacks, strokes, and peripheral arterial diseases.[199] Consequently, atherosclerosis presents a significant public health challenge. Key risk factors for atherosclerosis include aging, hypertension, smoking, physical inactivity, high cholesterol, obesity, and type 2 diabetes.[234]

Atherosclerosis is a chronic inflammatory condition triggered by the accumulation of plaques within major arteries such as the aorta, carotids, and femoral arteries. These plaques develop due to the buildup of fats, cholesterol, calcium, fibrous tissue, cells, and cellular waste.[234] Over time, this process results in the arteries narrowing and stiffening. As the plaque continues to develop, it can impede blood flow to vital organs and tissues, increasing the risk of various cardiovascular events, including heart attacks and strokes. Furthermore, in atherosclerosis, calcium deposits often form within the arterial walls, leading to calcification. This process contributes to the hardening of the arteries and further impedes blood flow.[235]

Research indicates that magnesium deficiency can influence lipoprotein metabolism, potentially contributing to atherosclerosis as a cardiovascular risk factor. Studies have shown that endothelial cells cultured in low magnesium environments activate nuclear factor-kappa beta, which, in turn, may initiate a cascade of cytokine responses[225]. Nuclear factor-kappa beta is important for controlling how the body responds to infections. When it's not regulated correctly, it can lead to various health issues like cancer, inflammatory diseases, autoimmune diseases, severe infections, and problems with the immune system's development.[236] Low magnesium levels in culture increases the endothelial cell secretion of RANTES (regulated on activation, normal T cell expressed and secreted), interleukin 8, and platelet-derived growth factor-BB, all of which play crucial roles in the development of atherogenesis (the process of forming plaques in the innermost layer of arteries). Furthermore, when endothelial cells are exposed to low levels of magnesium, they tend to increase the production of matrix metalloproteinase-2 and matrix metalloproteinase-9 along with their inhibitor, tissue inhibitor of metalloproteinases (TIMP-2).[225] Matrix metalloproteinase-2 (MMP-2) and matrix metalloproteinase-9 (MMP-9) are enzymes in the body that play a role in breaking down and remodeling the extracellular matrix, which is the structure that supports cells and tissues in the body. MMP-2 and MMP-9 are particularly important in processes like tissue repair, wound healing, and the remodeling of tissues during development. However, when their activity becomes excessive or uncontrolled, they can contribute to diseases such as cancer, arthritis, and cardiovascular disorders by breaking down healthy tissues excessively.[237] It is important to note that all these pathways lead to endothelial dysfunction by triggering the expression of inflammatory cytokines in the presence of magnesium deficiency.[225]

In rats subjected to a magnesium-deficient diet for a brief duration, several physiological changes are observed in their bodies. These changes include lower levels of magnesium, sphingomyelin (membrane phospholipid), high density lipoprotein (HDL), cholesterol and phosphatidylcholine:cholesterol ratio. Alongside reductions in tissue levels of glutathione, there is also evidence of leakage of cardiac enzymes like creatine kinase (CK) and lactic dehydrogenase (LDH). Additionally, there is activation of nitric oxide synthase (e-NOS and n-NOS) in all chambers of the heart. The changes in these parameters seem to happen more as the level of magnesium in the diet decreases. This can then lead to oxidative stress, which damages cells. Lower levels of glutathione and activation of e-NOS and N-NOS in various chambers of the heart are thought to contribute to early damage to the heart, which is marked by the release of CK and LDH enzymes.[238] Low magnesium levels might slow down the growth of endothelial cells and affect how they move. This happens because certain substances in the body decrease (CDC25B) while others increase (interleukin-1, vascular cell adhesion molecule-1, and plasminogen activator inhibitor-1) after magnesium deficiency. These changes lead to a pro-atherosclerotic state.[224]

In another animal study, it was observed that giving cholesterol-fed rabbits a magnesium-deficient diet significantly increased lipid buildup in their aortas.[239] Additionally, rabbits on this diet showed calcification in the inflamed areas of the aorta, as well as muscle fiber degeneration with inflammatory connective tissue growth in the cardiac muscle, stomach, and skeletal muscles.[239] This indicates that a magnesium-deficient diet can lead to atherosclerosis, aortic calcification, myocardial muscle fiber degeneration, and widespread inflammation. The study suggests that low magnesium intake exacerbates inflammation.

Treating patients with ischemic heart disease with magnesium for three months has been shown to increase the ratio of apolipoprotein A1 to apolipoprotein B by 13%.[240] Additionally, it reduces apolipoprotein B concentrations by 15% and lowers very-low-density lipoprotein concentrations by 27%.[240] Finally, magnesium therapy also tends to increase high-density lipoprotein levels. The authors of the study concluded: "magnesium deficiency might be involved in the pathogenesis of ischemic heart disease by altering the blood lipid composition in a way that disposes to atherosclerosis".[240] In kidney transplant recipients with low magnesium levels, supplementation with magnesium significantly reduces total cholesterol, low-density lipoprotein, and the ratio of total cholesterol to high-density lipoprotein.[241] It was also found that a lack of magnesium could worsen damage to the endothelial lining of blood vessels, which in turn promotes the development and advancement of atherosclerosis.[242]

Magnesium deficiency increases the risk of lipoprotein oxidation and the development of atherosclerosis.[217] In humans, prolonged magnesium deficiency has been linked to decreased serum magnesium levels, alongside elevated lipid and serum glucose levels. In young, seemingly healthy athletes, ongoing magnesium deficiency due to intense physical exertion was associated with sustained increases in cholesterol, triglycerides, and blood sugar levels over time.[243] More importantly, it was found that individuals in the intensive cardiac care unit have been observed to have low levels of magnesium in their blood mononuclear cells.[208] The authors concluded that the prevalence of intracellular magnesium deficiency among patients with cardiovascular disease is much higher than what serum magnesium levels would indicate. They emphasize that this deficiency may substantially contribute to the clinical morbidity associated with cardiovascular conditions.[208]

In conclusion, the collective findings of these studies indicate that magnesium supplementation may be beneficial as a therapeutic approach for the primary prevention of atherosclerosis.

Cardiomyopathy

Cardiomyopathy refers to a group of diseases that affect the heart muscle, leading to abnormalities in its structure and function. These conditions can impair the heart's ability to pump blood effectively to the rest of the body, potentially leading to symptoms such as fatigue, breathlessness, and swelling of the legs and abdomen. There are several types of cardiomyopathy, including dilated cardiomyopathy, hypertrophic cardiomyopathy, and restrictive cardiomyopathy, each characterized by specific changes in the heart muscle. While the exact cause of cardiomyopathy may vary depending on the type, common factors contributing to its development include genetic mutations, viral infections, high blood pressure, excessive alcohol consumption, and certain medications or toxins.[244]

Magnesium deficiency has been implicated in the cause of cardiomyopathy, as evidenced by both animal studies and research involving humans. In animal models, hamsters that were fed a diet lacking in magnesium developed cardiomyopathy characterized by areas of myocardial necrosis, calcification, and some infiltration of mononuclear and giant cells.[245] Furthermore, in hamsters administered nifedipine (a calcium channel blocker), there was a reduction in the abundance and diameter of lesions in a dose-dependent manner. Conversely, hamsters given digoxin (used to treat heart failure) exhibited a dose-dependent increase in lesion abundance and diameter. These findings lend support to the theory that the lesions stem from calcium overload following elevated myocardial sodium levels, which occur due to the inhibition of the Na^+–K^+–ATPase and subsequent sodium-calcium exchange in a state of magnesium deficiency.[245] The release of catecholamines are heightened during cellular magnesium depletion. The adverse effects resulting from the combination of catecholamine excess and magnesium deficiency have been observed to act synergistically in the myocardium. In rabbits, supplementation with magnesium has been shown to diminish the structural abnormalities associated with myocardial damage caused by epinephrine injection.[246]

In human studies, there is further evidence supporting the role of magnesium in cardiomyopathy. Individuals with hypoparathyroidism may develop cardiomyopathy, a condition that shows improvement with magnesium supplementation.[247] Moreover, cardiomyopathy and magnesium deficiency are frequently observed in individuals who engage in heavy alcohol consumption.[248] Additionally, it was shown that individuals living in low-magnesium equatorial regions, as well as those with a magnesium-deficient diet, can develop spontaneous endomyocardial fibrosis of undetermined etiology.[248-250]

From animal studies to human trials, magnesium supplementation has shown promising results in mitigating myocardial damage, improving cardiac function, and improving or reversing cardiomyopathy in some cases. Whether addressing magnesium deficiency in patients with specific medical conditions or as a preventive measure, incorporating adequate magnesium intake may offer significant benefits in combating cardiomyopathy.

Congestive Heart Failure

Congestive heart failure is a chronic condition characterized by the heart's inability to pump blood efficiently to meet the body's demands. As a result, fluid may accumulate in various parts of the body, leading to symptoms such as shortness of breath, fatigue, and swelling in the legs and abdomen. Congestive heart failure can develop gradually over time due to various underlying health conditions or acute events that affect the heart's function.[251] According to the World Health Organization, common causes of congestive heart failure include coronary artery disease, hypertension, valvular heart disease, myocardial infarction (heart attack), and cardiomyopathy.[252] These conditions can impair the heart's ability to pump effectively, leading to the onset and progression of congestive heart failure. Early detection, management of risk factors, and timely intervention are crucial in preventing and managing congestive heart failure, which remains a significant global health challenge.[251]

In individuals experiencing congestive heart failure, magnesium deficiency is frequently observed, stemming from various mechanisms.[44, 129, 253] Individuals with congestive heart failure might experience increased magnesium excretion in their urine due to diminished magnesium reabsorption in the kidney tubules. Certain medications, including diuretics and digoxin, can exacerbate this issue by reducing the reabsorption of magnesium in the kidney tubules.[88]

In individuals with heart failure, low magnesium levels also raise the risk of low potassium levels, potentially leading to ventricular arrhythmias and hemodynamic derangements (abnormalities or disturbances in the flow and pressure of blood within the cardiovascular system).[214] Magnesium depletion can worsen heart muscle function, heighten blood vessel constriction, and diminish cardiac energy reserves.[254] Additionally, magnesium deficiency has been linked to worse clinical outcomes in patients with congestive heart failure. It is important to note that micronutrient deficiency has been identified as an independent predictor of diminished health-related quality of life (HRQoL) and shortened cardiac event-free survival among patients diagnosed with heart failure (magnesium being an important micronutrient among them).[255]

Given that electrolyte imbalances are a common and potentially dangerous occurrence in individuals with heart failure, magnesium is believed to improve outcomes in congestive heart failure patients by preventing ventricular arrhythmias. In a randomized, double-blind, crossover trial conducted by Bashir et al. involving 21 patients with stable congestive heart failure due to coronary artery disease and receiving long-term loop diuretics, the impact of oral magnesium supplementation was investigated. Oral magnesium supplementation was found to reduce mean arterial pressure, systolic vascular resistance, and the frequency of isolated ventricular premature complexes, couplets, and non-sustained ventricular tachyarrhythmia.[256] Additionally, giving magnesium orotate (6,000 mg for 1 month, 3,000 mg for around 11 months) in a controlled, double-blind study involving 79 patients with severe congestive heart failure significantly improved the survival rate vs. placebo (75.7% vs. 51.6%, $p < 0.05$). Clinical symptoms improved in 38.5% of patients given magnesium orotate, whereas they deteriorated in 56.3% of patients given placebo ($p < 0.001$).[257]

However, further research is required to determine whether routine magnesium supplementation is justified for heart failure patients. Ralston et al. demonstrated that hypomagnesemia prevalence in ambulatory patients with dilated cardiomyopathy is relatively low (9%); nevertheless, magnesium primarily resides intracellularly (99%), leading to a weak association between serum magnesium levels and those in mononuclear cells, skeletal muscle cells, and cardiac muscle cells.[258]

Cardiac Arrhythmia

Cardiac arrhythmia, often referred to simply as arrhythmia, is a condition characterized by irregular heartbeats, either too fast, too slow, or irregular. These abnormalities in heart rhythm can disrupt the normal functioning of the heart, affecting its ability to pump blood effectively to the body. Arrhythmias can range from harmless to life-threatening and may occur in the atria (upper chambers) or ventricles (lower chambers) of the heart. Common causes of arrhythmias include coronary artery disease, high blood pressure, diabetes, smoking, excessive alcohol consumption, stress, electrolyte imbalances, and certain medications.[259]

The significance of magnesium supplementation in preventing arrhythmias among individuals with congestive heart failure has been well recognized. Insufficient magnesium levels may contribute to prolongation of the QT interval, ST-segment depression, and low amplitude T-waves.[260-262]

- **Prolongation of the QT interval:** This refers to a lengthening of the time it takes for the heart's electrical system to reset between beats, which can increase the risk of dangerous arrhythmias.[263]

- **ST-segment depression:** This indicates an abnormality in the part of the heart's electrical cycle that occurs between heartbeats, which can be a sign of reduced blood flow to the heart muscle.[263]

- **Low amplitude T-waves:** This means that the signals on the electrocardiogram (ECG) representing the recovery phase of the heart's electrical cycle are smaller than normal, suggesting potential issues with the heart's ability to recharge between beats.[263]

It is important to remember that magnesium plays a role in regulating the movement of various ions, including potassium, sodium, and calcium, across cell membranes. One notable association is between magnesium and potassium levels, where a deficiency in magnesium is frequently linked with a deficiency in potassium. In patients with congestive heart failure the use of thiazide diuretics can lead to depletion of both magnesium and potassium. This is especially true in those who need high doses of these diuretics.[264-267] Studies have demonstrated that even when serum potassium levels rise with repletion, the potassium level in muscle will not return to normal unless magnesium is replaced.[264, 268, 269] This underscores the critical role of magnesium depletion in increasing the risk of arrhythmias among patients with congestive heart failure. A recent prospective study further highlighted this association. They showed that among the 66% of patients with cardiac arrest who had magnesium abnormalities, none were successfully resuscitated.[270]

Supraventricular Tachycardia

Supraventricular tachycardia is a type of abnormal heart rhythm characterized by a rapid heartbeat originating above the heart's ventricles. Typically, supraventricular tachycardia involves electrical impulses that originate in the atria or the atrioventricular node, leading to a faster-than-normal heart rate. This condition can cause symptoms such as palpitations, dizziness, shortness of breath, and chest discomfort. Several factors can contribute to the development of supraventricular tachycardia, including abnormal electrical pathways in the heart, certain medical conditions like atrial fibrillation, underlying heart disease, electrolyte imbalances, excessive caffeine or alcohol consumption, stress, and certain medications.[271]

Many patients with supraventricular arrhythmias exhibit an intracellular magnesium deficiency, even when their serum magnesium levels appear normal. This discrepancy may explain the rationale for magnesium's benefits as an atrial antiarrhythmic agent.[272] Magnesium has been shown to improve atrial antiarrhythmic efficacy.[272] In a study by Maurat et al., they discovered that in vitro, experimental changes in atrial action potential can be triggered by a decrease in extracellular potassium or an overdose of digoxin. Elevating magnesium levels in the environment can rectify these alterations in atrial action potential. Magnesium appears to exert its effect through moderating the calcium inflow into the cell, a process exacerbated by low magnesium levels, rather than directly affecting Na+–K+–ATPase activity.[273] In the Framingham Heart Study, individuals with the lowest serum magnesium levels were found to have a 50% higher risk of developing atrial fibrillation compared to those with higher levels.[274] This association persisted even after excluding individuals taking diuretics. Thus, low serum magnesium levels are moderately associated with the onset of atrial fibrillation in individuals without pre-existing cardiovascular disease.[274] Furthermore, hypomagnesemia is prevalent in patients experiencing symptomatic atrial fibrillation, compounding the condition.[275] Addressing magnesium deficiency could offer benefits to those with symptomatic atrial fibrillation, particularly in individuals undergoing digoxin therapy.[275] Similarly, research by Lewis et al. indicated that magnesium treatment might lower the occurrence of ventricular ectopy (a type of arrhythmia or abnormal heart rhythm) in certain patients with chronic atrial fibrillation and mild to moderate hypomagnesemia who are receiving digoxin.[276]

In another investigation, seven patients diagnosed with congestive heart failure and undergoing long-term diuretic and digoxin therapy experienced idioventricular tachycardia. The administration of intravenous magnesium followed by intramuscular magnesium replenishment was noted to eliminate the arrhythmias.[277] Notably, five patients exhibited reduced lymphocyte magnesium and potassium levels despite having normal serum magnesium levels. This implies what we have stated numerous times; that normal serum magnesium does not guarantee sufficient magnesium levels throughout the body. A decline in cellular magnesium content increases susceptibility to digitalis-induced arrhythmias.[277]

Ventricular Arrhythmia

Ventricular arrhythmia encompasses a range of irregular heart rhythms originating from the heart's lower chambers, the ventricles. These abnormal rhythms disrupt the heart's ability to pump blood effectively, potentially leading to life-threatening complications. Ventricular arrhythmias can manifest as premature ventricular contractions (PVCs), ventricular tachycardia (VT), or ventricular fibrillation (VF). Causes of ventricular arrhythmias are diverse, including structural heart diseases such as coronary artery disease, myocardial infarction, heart failure, cardiomyopathies, and congenital heart defects. Additionally, electrolyte imbalances, medication side effects, and genetic factors can contribute to the development of ventricular arrhythmias.[278]

Magnesium treatment has demonstrated effectiveness in managing ventricular tachycardia. When conventional antiarrhythmic medications fail to control ventricular tachycardia and ventricular fibrillation, magnesium supplementation emerges as a viable therapeutic option.[279] Research suggests that magnesium-deficient dogs exhibit increased pressor sensitivity to epinephrine, requiring lower doses to trigger maximum pressor response. This underscores the potential role of magnesium in modulating cardiac rhythm disturbances. Dogs experiencing magnesium deficiency displayed a notably reduced threshold for initiating ventricular premature beats.[280] However, upon receiving magnesium supplementation, these dogs regained normal pressor sensitivity levels, effectively eliminating premature ventricular beats.[280] After magnesium infusions in humans, there was a notable increase in cellular potassium content, along with a significant decrease in the frequency of ventricular ectopic beats.[265]

Magnesium could be exerting its antiarrhythmic effects by preventing prolonged QTc intervals (reflects ventricular repolarization). In a study by Krasner et al. involving 24 patients scheduled for mitral valve replacement, it was observed that those who developed arrhythmias after surgery had not received pretreatment with oral magnesium. Additionally, they exhibited abnormal QTc intervals both before and after the operation.[281]

The role of intravenous magnesium supplementation has also been investigated in patients undergoing thrombolytic therapy for acute myocardial infarction. The experimental group receiving magnesium supplementation showed fewer ventricular arrhythmias compared to the control group, indicating that magnesium supplementation might serve as a safe and effective addition to thrombolytic therapy, potentially reducing short-term mortality and occurrences of ventricular arrhythmias post-acute myocardial infarction.[282] The association between magnesium depletion and severe ventricular arrhythmias like torsades de pointe has been well established. Papaceit et al. documented a case involving a patient with chronic magnesium depletion who developed torsades de pointes but showed significant improvement upon receiving magnesium supplementation.[283] However, magnesium supplementation has not demonstrated a reduction in implantable cardioverter-defibrillator (ICD) firing rates. It is important to note that the trial conducted was underpowered. Further prospective, large-scale, randomized controlled trials are necessary to better understand the impact of magnesium supplementation on ventricular arrhythmias in patients with ICDs.

Sudden Cardiac Death

Sudden cardiac death refers to an unexpected death from cardiac causes that occurs within one hour of symptom onset. It is a devastating event that can happen to individuals who may or may not have known pre-existing heart conditions. Sudden cardiac death is often caused by ventricular arrhythmias, such as ventricular fibrillation or ventricular tachycardia, which lead to an abrupt loss of heart function. While sudden cardiac death can occur in individuals of all ages, certain populations are at a higher risk, including those with a history of coronary artery disease, heart failure, cardiomyopathy, congenital heart defects, and arrhythmias.[284] According to the World Health Organization, sudden cardiac death accounts for a significant proportion of deaths worldwide, with estimates suggesting that approximately 17.9 million people die from cardiovascular diseases each year, making it the leading cause of death globally.[285]

Several studies spanning several decades have proposed a link between magnesium deficiency and sudden cardiac death. As mentioned in chapter two, evidence gathered from epidemiological, autopsy, clinical, and animal studies suggests a higher incidence of sudden cardiac death in regions with low magnesium levels in community water supplies. Moreover, individuals who succumbed to sudden cardiac death often exhibited low myocardial magnesium content. Sudden cardiac death secondary to magnesium deficiency may be secondary to cardiac arrhythmias and coronary artery vasospasm. Encouragingly, replenishing magnesium levels has shown promise in reducing the risk of arrhythmias and mortality following an acute myocardial infarction.[286]

Magnesium deficiency may contribute to sudden cardiac death through multiple mechanisms. Firstly, it makes the heart more vulnerable to the toxic effects of certain medications and oxygen deprivation. Thus, supplementing magnesium could offer significant protection to the heart. Secondly, as mentioned previously, magnesium activates a key enzyme called Na–K–ATPase, which can be inhibited by substances like lactate and free fatty acids during periods of reduced blood flow. Thirdly, magnesium deficiency may cause chronic electrical instability in the heart by disrupting the flow of sodium and calcium into heart cells.[287] A fourth potential mechanism involves the effect of hypomagnesaemia on vascular tone. In in-vitro laboratory experiments, researchers have observed that extracellular magnesium ions significantly influence the contractility and reactivities of blood vessels (arteries, arterioles, and veins) in various regional circulatory systems, across several mammalian species, including humans. Low levels of magnesium in the blood, known as hypomagnesemia, have been observed to heighten the contractile activity of various neurohumoral substances and to potentiate vasospasm. This effect is likely due to the regulation of calcium ion entry and distribution within cells. Coronary vasospasm has therefore been proposed as a potential mechanism contributing to sudden cardiac death.[288]

In further experiments, researchers isolated coronary arteries from dogs and subjected them to varying levels of magnesium in the surrounding fluid. They discovered that higher magnesium concentrations decreased the basal tension of the coronary arteries.

Conversely, a sudden reduction in magnesium led to increased contraction of both small and large coronary arteries.[289] Similarly, Altura's research revealed that reducing magnesium levels around perfused arterioles induced spontaneous vasoconstriction, heightened arteriolar resistance, tissue ischemia, and diminished venous outflow. Finally, when extracellular magnesium levels fall below normal, there is an increase in circulating vasoconstrictor hormones like angiotensin, serotonin, and acetylcholine.[290] The lower than normal extracellular magnesium levels may result in progressive vasoconstriction and vasospasm, leading to ischemia, which ultimately contributes to sudden cardiac death over time.

Strategies for increasing magnesium intake in an aim to reduce the risk of sudden cardiac death include dietary adjustments to include more magnesium-rich foods, adding magnesium to community water sources, fortifying foods with magnesium, and taking oral magnesium supplements.[286]

Coronary Vasospasm

Coronary vasospasm, also known as Prinzmetal's angina or variant angina, is a condition characterized by sudden, transient episodes of vasospasm in the coronary arteries, leading to temporary narrowing or complete occlusion of the blood vessels that supply the heart muscle with oxygen-rich blood. This phenomenon can result in chest pain (angina) and potentially life-threatening complications such as heart attack (myocardial infarction) or sudden cardiac death. While the exact cause of coronary vasospasm is not fully understood, certain risk factors and triggers have been identified. These include smoking, exposure to cold temperatures, emotional stress, cocaine use, and underlying conditions such as atherosclerosis or endothelial dysfunction. Additionally, abnormalities in the autonomic nervous system and imbalances in certain substances involved in blood vessel regulation, such as endothelin and nitric oxide, may contribute to the development of coronary vasospasm.[291]

Several studies have proposed a connection between insufficient magnesium levels and coronary artery spasms. Magnesium plays a crucial role in regulating the influx of calcium into smooth muscle cells, which is essential for smooth muscle contraction. Experiments conducted on dogs have shown that coronary arteries exposed to low magnesium solutions are more prone to vasospasm.[289] Furthermore, a decrease in magnesium levels can significantly increase the potential for contractile responses of both small and large arteries to norepinephrine.[289] Similar outcomes were observed in experiments involving intact dogs and isolated coronary arteries of pigs.[292, 293] In humans, low magnesium levels have been linked to variant angina, and measurement of erythrocyte magnesium content proves beneficial in gauging how easily vasospasm may occur.[294]

Guo et al. conducted a study assessing the intracellular and extracellular magnesium status in 12 women with variant angina. Their findings revealed a strong correlation between the 24-hour magnesium retention rate, intracellular magnesium concentrations in erythrocytes, and the severity of variant angina.[295] Teragawa et al. further demonstrated that magnesium infusion induces a non-site-specific basal coronary dilation and effectively suppresses acetylcholine-induced coronary spasms in patients diagnosed with vasospastic angina. Magnesium infusion proved effective in alleviating the intensity of chest pain and ST-segment deviations associated with coronary spasm. Following magnesium infusion, there was a notable improvement in the percent change in the diameter of spastic segments, shifting from -62.8±2.6% to -43.7±4.7% during coronary spasm.[296] These findings indicate the potential benefits of magnesium in managing symptoms among patients diagnosed with variant angina.

Thrombosis

Thrombosis refers to the formation of a blood clot within a blood vessel, obstructing the flow of blood through the circulatory system. This condition can occur in arteries or veins and poses significant health risks, including heart attack, stroke, and pulmonary embolism. Thrombosis typically arises due to a combination of factors, including abnormalities in blood flow, damage to blood vessel walls, and alterations in blood composition that promote clot formation. Common causes of thrombosis include prolonged immobility, surgery, trauma, obesity, smoking, hormonal changes (such as those occurring during pregnancy or with contraceptive use), certain medical conditions (such as cancer or autoimmune disorders), and genetic predispositions to clotting disorders.[297]

In various studies involving both animals and humans, magnesium deficiency has been associated with an increased tendency for blood clot formation, known as a prothrombotic state. For instance, in an uncontrolled study conducted in 1959 by Parsons et al., patients experiencing angina or myocardial infarction showed a remarkable decrease in mortality rates, from 30% to 1%, when they were treated with magnesium sulfate intramuscularly. This improvement was attributed to the beneficial effects of magnesium in reducing the inhibition of plasmin, an enzyme crucial for fibrinolysis, which is responsible for breaking down fibrin clots.[298] In a study conducted in 1986, it was found that bleeding time increased when magnesium was infused into patients with acute myocardial infarction.[299] Magnesium has been shown to inhibit ADP-induced platelet aggregation.[300] It has also been shown that treatment with magnesium infusion is effective in reducing certain clotting factors in patients with pre-eclampsia.[301]

In a study published in 1989, Paolisso et al. found that administering magnesium could alleviate platelet hypercoagulability in patients diagnosed with non-insulin-dependent diabetes.[302] Additionally, another researcher found that low intracellular magnesium levels contribute to platelet-dependent thrombosis in individuals with coronary artery disease.[226] These studies indicate that magnesium might be involved in reducing thrombosis, and supplementing with magnesium could be advantageous for specific groups of patients.

Mitral Valve Prolapse

Mitral valve prolapse is a heart condition characterized by the improper closing of the mitral valve, which separates the heart's left atrium and left ventricle. Instead of closing tightly, the valve's leaflets bulge (prolapse) upward into the atrium during the heart's contraction. Mitral valve prolapse is typically benign and may not cause symptoms or complications in many cases. The exact cause of mitral valve prolapse is often unclear, but it is believed to involve a combination of genetic factors and abnormalities in the structure of the valve or its supporting tissues. Additionally, certain conditions such as connective tissue disorders, Marfan syndrome, and Ehlers-Danlos syndrome may increase the risk of developing this condition.[303]

The precise mechanism behind mitral valve prolapse remains somewhat unclear. However, there is a suggestion that magnesium deficiency could be linked to the syndrome. A study comparing 49 individuals with mitral valve prolapse to a control group of similar age and gender found no significant difference in serum magnesium levels between the two groups. However, those with mitral valve prolapse exhibited lower levels of magnesium in their lymphocytes. These findings imply a potential association between lymphocyte magnesium deficiency and mitral valve prolapse.[304]

In another study conducted by Licholdziejewska et al, they compared serum magnesium levels in 141 individuals with severely symptomatic mitral valve prolapse to 40 healthy controls. Their findings revealed that a considerable number of patients with severe symptoms of mitral valve prolapse exhibited low serum magnesium levels.[305] Supplementation with magnesium resulted in alleviation of various symptoms such as chest pain, shortness of breath, weakness, palpitations, and anxiety, alongside a reduction in catecholamine excretion.[305] Despite these observations, further research is required to better understand the connection between magnesium deficiency and mitral valve prolapse syndrome.

Stroke

A stroke occurs when blood flow to a part of the brain is interrupted or reduced, depriving brain tissue of oxygen and nutrients. This leads to brain cell damage or death, resulting in loss of function controlled by that area of the brain, such as speech, movement, or memory. Strokes can be ischemic, caused by a blockage in an artery supplying blood to the brain, or hemorrhagic, caused by bleeding in the brain. The risk factors for stroke include high blood pressure, high cholesterol, smoking, obesity, diabetes, and physical inactivity.[306] According to the World Health Organization (WHO), stroke is a leading cause of death and disability worldwide, with approximately 6.2 million people dying from it annually. It is also a major cause of long-term disability, with millions of people left permanently disabled after surviving a stroke.[307]

Low levels of magnesium in the blood has been identified as a risk factor for cerebrovascular events and complications. Research conducted by Szabo et al. revealed that even a slight decrease in extracellular magnesium levels, from 1.2 to 0.8 mM, led to sustained relaxation of blood vessels when the endothelium was intact. However, when the endothelium was disrupted, this slight reduction in magnesium resulted in an increase in vascular tone. These findings suggest that magnesium influences human cerebral arterial tone through the action of an endothelium-derived relaxing factor rather than by directly altering smooth muscle tone. Furthermore, magnesium deficiency appears to contribute to endothelial dysfunction and subsequently to the development of atherosclerosis.[308]

Amighi et al. explored the prognostic significance of serum magnesium levels in relation to neurological events in patients with advanced atherosclerosis. They analyzed 323 patients with symptomatic peripheral artery disease and intermittent claudication. Compared to patients with the highest tertile of magnesium serum levels (>0.84 mmol/L), those with serum values <0.76 mmol/L (lowest tertile) showed a 3.29-fold increased adjusted risk (95% CI 1.34 to 7.90; p=0.009) for neurological events. However, patients with magnesium serum values ranging from 0.76 mmol/L to 0.84 mmol/L (middle tertile) did not exhibit an increased risk (adjusted HR 1.10; 95% CI 0.35 to 3.33; p=0.88). Therefore, there seems to be a correlation between decreased serum magnesium levels and an increased risk of neurological events (defined as ischemic stroke and/or carotid revascularization).[309] In another study encompassing 40 patients with acute ischemic strokes, there was an association between reduced serum magnesium levels and the severity of neurological impairment 48 hours post-stroke onset, as assessed by the National Institute of Health Stroke Scale (NIHSS). Furthermore, individuals with lower serum magnesium levels exhibited greater paresis (mild to moderate degree of muscular weakness) severity.[242]

In conclusion, these studies indicate the significant role that magnesium plays in the pathogenesis of acute ischemic stroke. Nonetheless, further research is required to better understand how magnesium influences the cerebral-vascular system and its mechanisms of action in this context.

Oxidative Stress and Myocardial Injury

Oxidative stress is a fundamental process in human physiology. It occurs when there's an imbalance between the production of reactive oxygen species and the body's ability to detoxify them or repair the resulting damage. Reactive oxygen species, such as superoxide radicals, hydrogen peroxide, and hydroxyl radicals, are natural byproducts of cellular metabolism and play essential roles in cell signaling and immune function. However, excessive reactive oxygen species production, often triggered by factors like environmental pollutants, unhealthy diet, or metabolic disorders, can overwhelm the body's antioxidant defenses.[310] In the myocardium, the heart muscle tissue, oxidative stress can lead to damage of lipids, proteins, and DNA, contributing to various cardiovascular diseases, including heart failure, atherosclerosis, and myocardial infarction. Additionally, oxidative stress is implicated in the aging process and the development of numerous chronic diseases across the body. It is important to understand the mechanisms of oxidative stress and its impact on cellular function so that we can mitigate its harmful effects and promote overall health and well-being.

Research indicates that magnesium deficiency plays a role in myocardial infarction via increased oxidative stress. This deficiency has been linked to an increase in the production of reactive oxygen species and cytokines, along with compromised vascular function in living organisms.[311] In addition, studies on various animal models have demonstrated that magnesium deficiency induces myocardial lesions. Rats that had been subjected to a magnesium-deficient diet exhibited reduced levels of superoxide dismutase and catalase (enzymes that protect cells from oxidative stress) in their hearts, resulting in diminished antioxidant defenses and heightened susceptibility to oxidative damage in the myocardium.[312] Hans et al. further illustrated that magnesium deficiency is associated with increased oxidative stress, marked by reductions in plasma antioxidants and elevated lipid peroxidation.[313] These findings suggest that the increased oxidative stress might stem from increased susceptibility of bodily organs to free radical damage.

In Syrian hamsters fed a magnesium-deficient diet, injury from oxidation (isoprenaline) significantly increased.[314] This observation underscores how magnesium deficiency amplifies the vulnerability of the cardiovascular system to oxidative harm. Similar trends were observed in human studies. Kharb and Singh estimated serum levels of malonaldehyde (MDA), magnesium, vitamin E, and total glutathione (GSH) in 22 patients with acute myocardial infarction alongside 15 healthy controls. Patients with acute myocardial infarction exhibited lower levels of magnesium, GSH, and vitamin E, along with elevated MDA levels.[315] These findings suggest that magnesium deficiency can exacerbate oxidative damage in post-ischemic myocardium.

Patients experiencing acute myocardial infarction often exhibit decreased magnesium levels, especially in the initial hours following the event. Urdal et al. conducted a study looking at mononuclear cell magnesium levels and magnesium retention post intravenous loading in patients with acute myocardial infarction compared to healthy volunteers. Interestingly, the study revealed that mononuclear cell magnesium concentrations before the magnesium retention test were slightly higher in patients with acute myocardial infarction compared to healthy volunteers, suggesting no significant magnesium depletion in the acute myocardial infarction group. However, when the magnesium retention test was conducted 4–11 days after admission in individuals with acute myocardial infarction, it was observed that the retention of magnesium amounted to 45±23% of the 30 mmol administered intravenously. (Retention exceeding 20% typically indicates magnesium deficiency.) The reason behind the increased retention of magnesium during the acute phase of myocardial infarction remains unclear. However, it is hypothesized that increased concentrations of circulating catecholamines during the early hours of myocardial infarction may contribute to this phenomenon.[316]

Rasmussen et al. also discovered that individuals with ischemic heart disease, both with and without acute myocardial infarction, exhibited significantly higher magnesium retention compared to the control group of healthy volunteers. This elevated magnesium retention indicates a state of magnesium deficiency among patients with ischemic heart disease. Notably, when the patients with ischemic heart disease were further categorized based on long-term diuretic treatment, those receiving such treatment displayed a 39% retention of magnesium (11.6mmol/L or 28.2mg/dL), whereas those not receiving diuretics showed a 29% retention (8.7mmol/L or 21.1mg/dL).[317] This study indicates that individuals with ischemic heart disease may experience significant magnesium deficiency, potentially exacerbated by long-term diuretic therapy. Additionally, research has demonstrated the beneficial impact of intravenous magnesium treatment in acute myocardial infarction, leading to reductions in both mortality rates and early cardiac insufficiency. Beyond its antiarrhythmic and vasodilatory effects, magnesium appears to shield cardiac cells from the detrimental effects of ischemia.[318]

Does Supplemental Calcium Increase Cardiovascular Risk?

In this section we are going to dive into the question of whether supplemental calcium intake poses an increased risk to cardiovascular health. While calcium supplementation is commonly advocated for bone health, recent studies have raised concerns about its potential impact on cardiovascular outcomes.

As women transition through perimenopause and into menopause there is often an increased focus on maintaining bone health due to the hormonal changes that occur during this stage of life. Calcium supplements have become a cornerstone in the management of bone health during perimenopause and menopause, primarily because of the heightened risk of osteoporosis and bone fractures associated with declining estrogen levels. Estrogen plays a crucial role in maintaining bone density by inhibiting bone resorption, and as estrogen levels decline during menopause, bone loss accelerates.[319] Consequently, women in this age bracket are more prone to developing osteoporosis, a condition characterized by weakened bones and an increased susceptibility to fractures.[319] To counteract this decline in bone density and reduce the risk of osteoporosis-related complications, healthcare providers often recommend calcium supplementation as part of a comprehensive approach to bone health management during perimenopause and menopause.

Meta-analyses of randomized controlled trials examining calcium supplementation, some including concurrent vitamin D intake, have revealed a modest increase in the risk of strokes and heart attacks among those receiving calcium supplements.[320] Whether these risks would be offset by taking a vitamin K2 and/or magnesium supplement should be determined, as vitamin K2 and magnesium help to keep calcium out of the arteries and into the bones. Recent observational studies within prospective cohorts have highlighted a potential link between supplemental calcium and heightened cardiovascular risk.[321-323] However, higher *dietary* calcium intake levels have been associated with cardiovascular protection or have shown neutral outcomes in terms of cardiovascular health.[321, 322, 324] Furthermore, there are theoretical reasons to anticipate that optimal calcium nutrition might safeguard vascular health. Diets rich in calcium have been shown to reduce the secretion of parathyroid hormone. It's worth noting that even mild secondary hyperparathyroidism, common in the elderly, is thought to elevate cardiovascular risk.[325, 326] A significant intake of calcium also typically inhibits the absorption of dietary phosphate by forming an insoluble complex with it. Recent findings indicate that elevated phosphate intake may increase cardiovascular risk, even among individuals with normal kidney function.[327] Surprisingly, high calcium intakes (from diet and supplements) have not been correlated with an increased risk of vascular calcification.[328] It's possible that including dietary calcium intake with calcium supplementation may have masked this potential issue. However, research has examined the immediate vascular effects of a slight increase in serum calcium levels following an oral dose of calcium citrate; compared to a placebo, individuals in the calcium group experienced a decrease in arterial stiffness and an improvement in myocardial perfusion.[329] However, acute effects cannot necessarily tell us long-term effects. Nevertheless, individuals who received calcium supplementation did not experience as significant a decrease in blood pressure during the day, and there was an increase in a coagulation index, suggesting that taking calcium supplements may increase blood clotting.

The heightened risk of vascular events linked to calcium supplementation in certain controlled studies has been criticized. Indeed, the studies that reported increased cardiovascular events with calcium supplementation were not the primary endpoint of the study. A randomized trial comparing calcium carbonate supplementation (1,200 mg per day) with placebo evaluating the risk of vascular events and mortality as a primary end point did not show a higher risk of death or first-time hospitalization from atherosclerotic vascular disease compared with placebo.[330, 331] One author concluded, "In summary, when patients are randomized and cardiovascular events are carefully adjudicated, there is no compelling evidence that calcium supplementation increases the rate of major cardiovascular events. Earlier trials may have had unforeseen ascertainment bias, causing the perception of an increase in cardiovascular events."[330] Additional randomized controlled trials where cardiovascular events are the primary endpoint should be performed to fully ascertain the benefits and risks of calcium supplementation.

It is important to consider the likelihood that in certain individuals, elevated intake of supplemental calcium might disrupt magnesium balance.[7] Recent epidemiological evidence, including meta-analyses, strongly suggests that increased dietary magnesium intake or higher serum magnesium levels correlate with a decreased risk of vascular events such as arrhythmias, diabetes, hypertension, metabolic syndrome, vascular calcification, and mortality.[332, 333] While these findings may partly stem from the advantages of consuming nutrient-dense whole foods rather than solely magnesium itself, magnesium frequently emerges as protective even after conducting multiple regression analyses attempting to account for this factor. Furthermore, as we have seen, short-term studies into magnesium supplementation among individuals at increased cardiovascular risk have frequently revealed protective effects, especially among those with initially low magnesium levels. Notably, among individuals with coronary artery disease, administering magnesium supplements reduces ex vivo platelet-dependent thrombosis, enhances flow-mediated vasodilation of the brachial artery, improves exercise tolerance, VO2max, and left ventricular ejection fraction during exercise.[226, 334-337] In a meta-analysis of placebo-controlled studies assessing the effects of supplemental magnesium on hypertensive individuals with baseline systolic pressure exceeding 155 mmHg, there was a notable decrease of 18.7 mmHg in systolic pressure and 10.9 mmHg in diastolic pressure, both statistically significant.[232] The precise mechanism underlying the observed benefits of optimal magnesium levels warrants additional investigation, although it is hypothesized that magnesium counteracts certain pro-inflammatory effects associated with elevated cytoplasmic calcium levels.[338, 339]

Magnesium is sometimes referred to as 'nature's calcium blocker' in certain contexts.[340] This designation stems from its role in intracellular concentrations, where magnesium competes with calcium for binding to proteins like calmodulin and other 'EF-hand' calcium-binding proteins. As a result, when magnesium binds to these proteins, they assume an 'off' configuration.[338, 339] Furthermore, having adequate magnesium levels and intake seems to mitigate the risk of vascular calcification, which is important particularly since epidemiological studies link calcium supplement usage to increased risk of coronary calcification.[323, 333, 341, 342]

In forthcoming epidemiological investigations, it would be prudent to categorize calcium supplement users based on whether they concurrently use magnesium supplements and to assess their dietary magnesium intake. Meanwhile, individuals, particularly those with relatively refined diets, considering calcium supplementation might find it beneficial to opt for a supplement containing highly absorbable magnesium as well, aiming for a balanced 2:1 ratio of calcium to magnesium in their overall dietary intake (e.g., 1,000-1,200 mg calcium/500-600 mg magnesium). We will cover more about dietary calcium and magnesium balance in chapter 7.

Conclusion

In short, magnesium plays a crucial role in cardiovascular health. It is instrumental for maintaining cellular membrane potential, facilitating mitochondrial function, and actively participating in the body's antioxidant pathways. Consequently, magnesium deficiency can result in severe morbidity and mortality, and it has been linked to various cardiovascular ailments including hypertension, cardiomyopathy, cardiac arrhythmia, atherosclerosis, dyslipidemia, and diabetes. Regrettably, the Western diet (standard American diet) often lacks adequate magnesium due to the refinement and processing of foods. In addition, hypomagnesemia frequently goes undiagnosed in hospitalized patients. Ultimately what we can conclude and what we should be prioritizing is optimizing magnesium status through dietary interventions or supplementation. This may hold promise in mitigating cardiovascular risk factors and improving overall cardiovascular health.

Chapter 4 - Magnesium and Brain Health

Magnesium is considered the "master mineral." It is a key element essential for the proper functioning of the human body. Beyond its well-known role in maintaining bone health, muscle function, and heart rhythm, magnesium also significantly impacts the complex operations of the brain. This mineral plays a crucial role in numerous biochemical processes within the brain, affecting everything from neurotransmitter regulation to synaptic plasticity.[343]

At the most fundamental level, and as we have mentioned, magnesium serves as a cofactor for over 600 enzymatic reactions in the body, many of which are integral to brain function.[2] One of its primary functions in the brain is its involvement in the regulation of neurotransmitters, the chemical messengers that facilitate communication between neurons. Magnesium modulates the activity of neurotransmitter receptors, including those for glutamate and gamma-aminobutyric acid (GABA), thereby influencing synaptic transmission and neuronal excitability.[343]

Moreover, magnesium plays a crucial role in maintaining the integrity of the blood-brain barrier, a selectively permeable membrane that protects the brain from harmful substances circulating in the bloodstream. By regulating the tight junctions between endothelial cells in the blood vessels of the brain, magnesium helps safeguard the delicate neural tissue from potential damage.[343]

The interaction between magnesium and the brain extends beyond the basic cellular processes that impact cognitive function, mood regulation, and the stress response. Research suggests that magnesium deficiency may play a key role in cognitive decline, mood disorders, an increased risk of neurological disorders as well as neurodegenerative conditions like Alzheimer's and Parkinson's disease.[343, 344]

Magnesium has garnered attention for its potential therapeutic benefits in addressing a wide range of brain disorders. Many of these will be covered in the following pages. As we dive deeper into the intricate interplay between magnesium and the brain, we will explore its implications for various neurological conditions, spanning from migraine and mood disorders to sleep disorders and neurodegenerative diseases. By unraveling the mechanisms underlying magnesium's influence on brain health and function, we aim to uncover new avenues for therapeutic intervention and enhance your understanding of the intricate complexities of the human brain.

Sleep Disorders

Sleep is often regarded as the cornerstone of good health and well-being. It eludes many individuals worldwide, with sleep disorders posing a significant public health concern. In today's fast-paced society, characterized by constant connectivity and demanding schedules, the prevalence of sleep disturbances has reached alarming levels, impacting individuals of all ages and demographics.

Statistics reveal a staggering prevalence of sleep disorders, with approximately 1 in 3 adults experiencing occasional insomnia, and up to 10% to 30% suffering from chronic insomnia.[345] Beyond insomnia, sleep apnea, restless leg syndrome, narcolepsy, and other sleep-related conditions afflict millions, disrupting the natural rhythm of sleep and impairing overall quality of life.[346]

The ramifications of untreated sleep disorders extend far beyond individual discomfort, imposing substantial economic burdens on society. Globally, the societal costs associated with sleep disorders, including healthcare expenses, lost productivity, and accidents, amount to over $94 billion annually.[346] Moreover, the toll on public health is compounded by the morbidity and mortality linked to sleep disturbances, with increased risks of cardiovascular disease, diabetes, obesity, and mental health disorders.[346]

Amidst the escalating prevalence and profound impact of sleep disorders, the search for safe and effective interventions remains paramount. In recent years, growing interest has emerged in the potential role of magnesium as a natural remedy for sleep disturbances. Magnesium has garnered attention for its ability to modulate neurotransmitter pathways, regulate stress response, and promote relaxation.[347]

Preliminary research suggests that magnesium deficiency may contribute to sleep disturbances, highlighting the importance of adequate magnesium intake for optimal sleep quality. Furthermore, supplementation with magnesium has shown promise in improving sleep latency, duration, and quality, without the side effects commonly associated with traditional sleep medications.[348]

As we navigate the complex landscape of sleep disorders and their societal impact, exploring the potential of magnesium as a safe and effective intervention offers hope for addressing this pervasive health challenge. In the following sections, we will investigate the mechanisms underlying magnesium's influence on sleep, examine the evidence supporting its efficacy, and consider its implications for promoting restorative sleep and enhancing overall well-being.

Insomnia

Insomnia is characterized as the persistent difficulty initiating or maintaining sleep. It is a prevalent sleep disorder that profoundly impacts the lives of those affected. Individuals with insomnia typically experience restless nights, marked by frequent awakenings, difficulty falling asleep, or waking up too early and being unable to return to sleep.[349] The consequences of insomnia extend beyond mere fatigue, as it can lead to daytime impairment, diminished cognitive function, mood disturbances, and overall reduced quality of life.[350] The relentless cycle of sleeplessness can exacerbate stress, anxiety, and depression, further compounding the challenges faced by individuals struggling to attain restorative sleep. Insomnia not only disrupts nightly routines but also permeates into daily activities, affecting productivity, relationships, and emotional well-being.[348] Insomnia, being one of the most prevalent sleep disorders globally, demands careful attention to help those affected in restoring restful sleep.[345]

Insomnia can become more common as people age, though it is not an unavoidable part of getting older. Many elderly individuals, without specific geriatric conditions, may struggle with significant sleep problems. These include changes such as shorter sleep duration, reduced sleep efficiency (the percentage of time spent asleep after going to bed), and decreased deep sleep, all of which fall under the category of insomnia. Studies have shown that insomnia affects a significant portion of the population, with rates ranging from 10% to 48% across different age groups.[345] Among the elderly, around 40-50% of those aged 60 and above are estimated to experience insomnia.[350]

Aging poses a significant risk for magnesium deficiency, with several changes occurring in magnesium levels as individuals grow older. Magnesium levels decrease due to a decline in bone mass, which serves as a major magnesium source in the body.[351] Despite the vital role magnesium plays in bodily functions, studies indicate that many societies, including certain groups of elderly people, have inadequate dietary magnesium intake.[1] This deficiency may stem from numerous health conditions, a decrease in the magnesium content of our food and a tendency to consume more processed foods.[1, 350] Interestingly, while magnesium requirements remain unchanged with age, aging is associated with alterations in magnesium metabolism, including reduced intestinal absorption and increased excretion through urine and feces, which is often exacerbated by medication use.[351] Notably, reduced magnesium intake emerges as a key contributor to this age-related magnesium deficiency.[2]

Magnesium plays a crucial role in the conductivity of ion channels, such as the N-Methyl-D-aspartic acid receptor and the activation of potassium channels. The N-methyl-D-aspartate receptor is a receptor of glutamate, the primary excitatory neurotransmitter in the human brain.[350] Magnesium inhibits this neurotransmitter thereby promoting muscle relaxation. Additionally, magnesium is vital for the binding of neurotransmitters like dopamine, serotonin, and norepinephrine to their receptors. It has been shown that magnesium also plays a role in the regulation of gamma-aminobutyric acid (GABA), potentially aiding in inducing calmness and serving as a sedative to support sleep. GABA is a key inhibitory neurotransmitter in the central nervous system that counteracts the excitatory effects of glutamate, through reducing the release of glutamate from presynaptic neurons.[352] As a natural antagonist of N-methyl-D-aspartate receptors and an agonist of GABA, magnesium appears to be pivotal in the regulation of sleep and modulating sleep patterns.[350]

In a double-blind randomized clinical trial, 46 elderly subjects were randomly assigned to either 500 mg of magnesium or a placebo daily for 8 weeks. It was concluded that supplementation with magnesium appears to improve various aspects of insomnia in older individuals. These include subjective measures such as the Insomnia Severity Index score (screening tool for insomnia), sleep efficiency, duration of sleep, time taken to fall asleep, and instances of early morning awakening. Additionally, magnesium supplementation was shown to positively affect objective measures of insomnia, such as the concentration of serum renin, melatonin, and serum cortisol. These findings indicate that magnesium supplementation significantly improves both subjective and objective aspects of sleep and could be beneficial for addressing sleep issues in older adults.[350]

Low levels of magnesium in the body have been linked to various health conditions that involve ongoing inflammation and stress.[353] Some research in animals suggests that not getting enough magnesium, similar to what often happens in humans, might make inflammation or stress worse, especially if sleep is disrupted.[354] To investigate this, a study was conducted with 100 adults (22 men and 78 women) aged between 59 to 85 years old who had poor sleep quality. They were split into two groups, with one group taking a magnesium citrate supplement (320mg) and the other group taking a placebo for seven weeks. Based on food diaries, it was found that over half of the participants consumed less magnesium than the Estimated Average Requirement (EAR) for magnesium. This was associated with higher body mass index (BMI) and inflammation levels.[354] Despite this, most participants showed improvements in sleep quality and increased magnesium levels in their red blood cells, regardless of whether they took a magnesium supplement or a placebo. However, those who had low magnesium levels in their blood at the start of the study saw an increase in their blood magnesium levels only with magnesium supplementation. In addition, the supplement reduced inflammation (c-reactive protein) in those who had high inflammation levels at the beginning of the study. The authors concluded, "The findings show that many individuals have a low magnesium status associated with increased chronic inflammatory stress that could be alleviated by increased magnesium intake".[354]

Melatonin is a hormone produced and secreted by the pineal gland. It helps regulate our circadian rhythm (body's internal clock), which controls various functions such as sleep patterns. Melatonin levels are normally highest at night and lowest during the day. Studies in animals and humans show that melatonin attaches to receptors in the brain, helping to promote sleep and adjust our sleep schedule.[355]

It has been suggested that low magnesium levels are associated with reduced melatonin and magnesium supplementation increases the activity of serotonin N-acetyltransferase, an enzyme involved in making melatonin.[355] A small study investigated the impact of a magnesium-deficient diet on plasma melatonin in male rats. The results showed that rats on the magnesium-deficient diet had significantly lower melatonin levels compared to those with adequate magnesium levels.[356]

In another study, the effects of magnesium were examined on the sleep-wake cycle. The sleep-wake cycle, also known as the circadian rhythm, is your body's internal clock that regulates when you feel tired and when you feel awake. Two groups of rats were compared. One group was kept on a magnesium-deficient diet for 9 weeks, while the other group was initially fed a magnesium-deficient diet for 7 weeks followed by a normal diet for 4 weeks. The magnesium-deficient diet led to changes in sleep patterns and brain activity, with increased wakefulness and reduced slow-wave sleep (deep sleep) after 6-7 weeks. Sleep became disorganized after 9 weeks, indicating heightened neuronal excitability. However, reintroducing magnesium restored normal sleep patterns and brain activity.[357]

The research highlights the significant role of magnesium in regulating sleep patterns and brain activity. Given these findings, ensuring sufficient magnesium intake may offer a promising avenue for managing insomnia and improving overall sleep quality.

Restless Leg Syndrome

Restless Legs Syndrome is a prevalent condition affecting approximately 7–10% of adults in North America.[358] It is characterized by four main clinical features outlined by The Restless Legs Syndrome Foundation. These include an urge to move the legs, typically accompanied by uncomfortable sensations, symptoms worsening during periods of rest, relief through movement, and worsening symptoms in the evening or at night.[358] Periodic leg movements in sleep occur in around 80% of individuals with restless leg syndrome.[359] Both genetic and environmental factors contribute to the prevalence and severity of restless leg syndrome, with iron deficiency, pregnancy, and renal failure among the influencing factors. Restless leg syndrome has been associated with poor sleep and reduced quality of life.[359]

Emerging evidence suggests that oral magnesium therapy could provide relief for patients experiencing moderate restless legs syndrome. A study involving 10 patients with insomnia related to periodic leg movements in sleep or mild-to-moderate restless legs syndrome looked at the effects of oral magnesium administration over 4–6 weeks.

After magnesium supplementation, there was a significant decrease in periodic leg movements associated with arousals, along with a moderate reduction in periodic leg movements without arousal.[360] Additionally, sleep efficiency notably improved. These findings suggest that magnesium treatment may offer a beneficial alternative therapy for mild to moderate restless legs syndrome or periodic leg movements-related insomnia.[360]

Another paper presented findings from a study involving ten individuals with restless legs syndrome, focusing solely on restless legs syndrome related factors and excluding other neuropsychiatric conditions.[361] Polysomnographic recordings (sleep study) over 8 hours revealed significant disturbances in sleep organization, characterized by restless sleep with frequent nocturnal awakenings. As seen in other parasomnias linked to magnesium deficiency, disruptions in sleep patterns were observed, including restless sleep, heightened light slow wave sleep, and reduced REM sleep duration.[361] These findings underscore the potential role of magnesium deficiency in restless legs syndrome related sleep disturbances and highlight the need for further research in this area.

Sleep Apnea

Human beings spend roughly one-third of their lives sleeping, highlighting the vital role of restful sleep in maintaining overall health. However, functional disorders like obstructive sleep apnea can disrupt sleep patterns, leading to decreased quality of life and increased health risks. Obstructive sleep apnea is characterized by recurrent episodes of upper airway collapse during sleep, often caused by anatomical and non-anatomical factors.[362] Respiratory airflow can be disrupted when the tongue and surrounding soft tissues fall back into the throat, creating a physical blockage, typically due to the effects of gravity and muscle relaxation.[362] Symptoms of obstructive sleep apnea can range from snoring and daytime sleepiness to memory loss and irritability. Left untreated, obstructive sleep apnea can significantly impact a person's quality of life.

A systematic review and meta-analysis of six studies found four important take aways.[363] First, individuals with obstructive sleep apnea tend to have lower serum magnesium levels compared to healthy individuals, despite their levels falling within the normal range. Second, obstructive sleep apnea patients are more prone to magnesium deficiency. Third, the severity of obstructive sleep apnea appears to inversely impact serum magnesium levels, with higher Apnea-Hypopnea Index (index used to indicate the severity of sleep apnea) scores correlating with lower magnesium levels. Fourth, serum magnesium levels in these patients show associations with various biomarkers linked to cardiovascular disease risks, such as C-reactive protein (inflammatory marker), ischemia-modified albumin (sensitive and early biochemical marker of ischemia), and carotid intima-media thickness (measure used to diagnose the extent of carotid atherosclerotic vascular disease).[363] Additionally, magnesium levels may potentially correlate with biomarkers related to lipid profiles, glucose metabolism, calcium, and heavy metals.[363]

According to their research and the literature reviewed, these authors concluded that obstructive sleep apnea induces sleep deprivation, which elevates oxidative stress levels.[363] Magnesium, essential for antioxidant enzyme activity like superoxide dismutase, is consequently depleted due to increased oxidative stress.[364] This imbalance disrupts the magnesium balance and can exacerbate chronic systemic inflammation, raising the risk of metabolic, endocrine, and cardiovascular disorders.[364] Insufficient dietary intake further compounds the decline in magnesium levels.

It was concluded that individuals with obstructive sleep apnea are prone to low magnesium levels and enhancing these levels could potentially aid in treating both obstructive sleep apnea and magnesium deficiency.[363] While further research is warranted to confirm these findings, it appears that magnesium supplementation may benefit obstructive sleep apnea patients.

Magnesium emerges as a promising mineral in the realm of sleep disorders and offers a wide range of benefits. Not only can magnesium supplementation alleviate symptoms associated with sleep disorders, but it can also address underlying deficiencies that may exacerbate these conditions. By addressing both the symptoms and underlying deficiencies, magnesium offers a holistic approach to improving sleep quality and overall well-being. As mentioned, further studies are needed, specifically looking at the mechanisms of magnesium's effects on sleep disorders. Magnesium has been shown to be a safe and effective intervention for individuals seeking relief from sleep-related challenges.

Mood Disorders

Mood disorders encompass a wide range of mental health conditions, including anxiety, stress, depression, bipolar disorder, schizophrenia, and attention-deficit/hyperactivity disorder (ADHD). These disorders affect millions of people globally and pose significant challenges to individuals, families, and societies as a whole. In the United States alone, mood disorders are highly prevalent, with millions of adults and children experiencing the debilitating effects of these conditions.[365]

Approximately one in five Americans grapple with mental health issues, with mood disorders representing a significant portion of these issues. Recent estimates suggest that approximately 20.9 million adults in the United States, aged 18 and above, contend with mood disorders.[365, 366] Research underscores the significant impact of mood disorders, indicating that approximately 9.7% of American adults experience a mood disorder each year.[366] Notably, the prevalence of mood disorders tends to be higher among females, affecting around 11.6%, compared to males, affecting approximately 7.7%. Moreover, it's projected that approximately 21.4% of adults will confront a mood disorder at some point in their lives.[365] The prevalence of ADHD is between 5% and 10% in children, while it is estimated to be around 4% amongst adults.[367]

The economic burden of mood disorders extends far beyond the direct costs of treatment and healthcare services. Lost productivity is a significant issue, as individuals with mood disorders often experience impairments in cognitive function, concentration, and decision-making abilities, leading to absenteeism in the workplace.[368] Severe cases can result in disability, necessitating financial support through disability benefits and social welfare programs. Additionally, family members and caregivers bear a substantial burden, both emotionally and financially, as they provide care and support.[368] Comorbidities with other medical conditions further strain healthcare systems and increase healthcare expenditures. Moreover, individuals with untreated mood disorders are at higher risk of involvement with the criminal justice system, adding to the economic burden through incarceration and rehabilitation costs.[350] Addressing these economic challenges requires comprehensive strategies focused on early intervention, access to mental healthcare services, and efforts to reduce stigma surrounding mental illness.

Beyond the economic impact, mood disorders contribute to significant morbidity and mortality rates. Individuals with untreated mood disorders are at higher risk for substance abuse, self-harm, and suicide. Suicide is a leading cause of death worldwide, with depression being a major risk factor.[369]

While the treatment landscape for mood disorders includes various pharmaceutical and therapeutic interventions, emerging research suggests that magnesium may offer potential benefits in helping with these conditions. Magnesium is involved in numerous biochemical processes in the body, including neurotransmitter regulation and stress response. [370] While some of the precise mechanisms are still being researched, magnesium supplementation has shown promise in reducing symptoms associated with mood disorders and improving overall mental well-being.[370]

We'll look at common mood disorders and examine the role of magnesium in their pathophysiology and therapeutic applications. By understanding the connection between magnesium and mood disorders, we hope to shed light on novel approaches to enhancing mental health and improving the lives of those affected by these conditions.

Anxiety and Stress Disorders

Anxiety and stress disorders are pervasive challenges affecting individuals across all walks of life. Characterized by overwhelming feelings of worry, fear, and apprehension, these disorders can significantly impact one's emotional well-being and daily functioning.[371] Stress and anxiety affects nearly everyone at some point in their lives. In today's fast-paced and demanding society, the prevalence of these disorders is on the rise.[371] According to the American Institute of Stress, 75% to 90% of doctor visits have a stress-related component.[372] Stress impacts both mental and physical health, triggering changes like increased blood pressure, heart rate, respiration, anxiousness and alertness. This can also potentially lead to long-term issues such as cognitive impairments and memory disorders, depending on its duration and nature.[372] However, emerging research suggests that magnesium may offer relief for those struggling with anxiety and stress.

Stress is often viewed as a psychological response to external pressures. From a neurobiological standpoint, stress serves as an adaptive system that continually evaluates and interacts with the environment. An overload of this system can lead to negative health consequences.[373] Magnesium, a crucial nutrient for human health, is commonly deficient in the general population. This deficiency, given magnesium's role in numerous bodily functions, can heighten the risk of both physical and mental health disorders over time. Notably, symptoms of magnesium deficiency closely resemble those of stress, including fatigue, irritability, and mild anxiety.[69]

Studies have revealed a link between stress-related symptoms like anxiety and autonomic dysfunction with magnesium deficiency. Stressful situations, both mental and physical, lead to increased magnesium excretion from the body, exacerbating stress responses.[374] Paradoxically, magnesium deficiency worsens the body's reaction to stress. It has been shown that compensating for magnesium deficiency enhances the nervous system's ability to withstand stress. However, as has been mentioned, diagnosing magnesium deficiency poses challenges, as blood magnesium levels may remain constant due to release from bone tissue.[374]

In the early 1990s, Galland and Seelig introduced the concept of a two-way relationship between magnesium and stress, often referred to as the "vicious cycle."[70, 120] As mentioned, this concept suggests that stress can lead to magnesium loss, causing a deficiency, which in turn increases the body's susceptibility to stress. The adrenergic impacts of psychological stress triggers a transfer of magnesium from inside the cells to outside, leading to higher excretion through urine and eventual depletion of bodily reserves.[120] Initially, this shift of magnesium has a protective role.[375] Normally, magnesium helps calm the brain by reducing excitatory signals (glutamate) and promoting GABA activity, resulting in an inhibitory effect.[376] It also helps reduce the body's response to stress hormones such as epinephrine, adrenaline and cortisol.[376] However, as mentioned, long term chronic stress and anxiety can deplete magnesium levels. This ongoing loss can compromise magnesium's calming effect and lead to overactivity in the brain's stress response system.[344] It is important to note that the relationship between stress and magnesium has been widely studied in both animals and humans.

Shedding light on how stress hormones impact magnesium levels and their clinical implications, Whyte et al. examined the influence of adrenaline infusion on plasma magnesium levels. Their findings revealed a significant decrease in magnesium levels during the infusion time, as well as an hour after the infusion ended, with no signs of recovery.[377] Various studies have shown that stress exposure affects both serum and urine magnesium levels. A study on young adults exposed to chronic or sub-chronic stressors documented notable decreases in plasma and total magnesium concentrations over three months.[378] During an examination period, university students experienced heightened anxiety, coinciding with an elevation in urinary magnesium excretion.[379] Similarly, in a study involving college students during a month-long examination period, with heightened stress and anxiety levels, there was a significant decrease in erythrocyte magnesium levels.[102] Mocci et al. who studied the effect of noise on catecholamines and magnesium levels in the serum as well as urinary excretions on healthy men found variations in blood and urine magnesium levels. Interestingly, serum magnesium increased shortly after noise exposure, while urine excretion of magnesium peaked within hours and lasted up to two days.[380]

Magnesium ions have been found to regulate the activity of the hypothalamic-pituitary adrenocortical axis, which is the primary system involved in responding to stress.[381] Activation of the hypothalamic-pituitary adrenocortical axis through corticotropin releasing hormone leads to various physiological, hormonal, and behavioral changes during stress, often manifesting as symptoms of anxiety.[382] Disruptions of the corticotropin releasing hormone and hypothalamic-pituitary adrenocortical axis have been proposed to contribute to pathological anxiety.[383] In a study by Sartori et al. they looked at how a lack of magnesium in the diet affects anxiety levels and the body's stress response in mice. They found that mice with low magnesium levels displayed more signs of anxiety compared to those with normal levels.[384] Interestingly, when they treated these mice with antidepressants or anti-anxiety medications, their anxiety improved. This study suggests that low magnesium levels may lead to increased anxiety and alterations in how the hypothalamic-pituitary adrenocortical axis responds to stress.

Research on the microbiome-gut-brain axis highlights the bidirectional relationship between the gut microbiota and the brain. Nowadays there is substantial evidence connecting anxiety and depression disorders to the microbial community residing in the

94

gastrointestinal system.[385] A study looked at a six-week magnesium deficient diet on both gut microbiota composition and anxiety-like behavior in mice, and investigated any potential correlation between the two.[386] Findings revealed a significant correlation between gut microbiota composition and the behavior of mice on the magnesium-deficient diet. This dietary deficiency led to alterations in gut microbiota and was linked to changes in anxiety-like behavior.[386]

Human studies consistently support animal findings, showing a correlation between low magnesium levels and stress or depression. Akarachkova et al. examined Russian women with chronic emotional stress and found that 60% had magnesium deficiency, alongside symptoms like irritability and fatigue.[387] Other studies revealed subclinical magnesium deficiency in up to 45% of stressed and anxious individuals.[388] Nielsen et al. discovered that among 96 American adults with sleep disorders, often associated with stress, 58% had low magnesium intake and higher C-reactive protein levels (a marker of inflammation).[354] Additionally, chronic stress, anxiety and magnesium deficiency may heighten vulnerability to depressive disorders.[389]

Research has consistently shown that magnesium affects various critical physiological processes involved in responding to stress and anxiety. Some of these include:

- Magnesium helps serotonin work better by improving its connection to its receptor on cell membranes.[390] Serotonin, a neurotransmitter, communicates messages between nerve cells in both your brain (central nervous system) and your body (peripheral nervous system). It also supports the production of serotonin by assisting an enzyme called tryptophan hydroxylase.[390]

- Magnesium blocks glutamate (excitatory neurotransmitter) activity both directly, by inhibiting the glutamate N-methyl-D-aspartate receptor, and indirectly, by promoting its reuptake into synaptic vesicles through the stimulation of the sodium-potassium ATPase. This prevents its excessive activation.[376]

- Magnesium indirectly lowers adrenocorticotropic hormone release by influencing neurotransmission pathways, thereby reducing cortisol levels in the body.[69, 376, 384]   Furthermore, long-term magnesium supplementation lowers 24-hour urinary cortisol levels.[391]

- Magnesium enhances gamma-aminobutyric acid (GABA) transmission by acting as an agonist, increasing gamma-aminobutyric acid (GABA) levels. It binds to and activates GABA receptors in the brain, effectively slowing down brain activity.[376]

- Magnesium likely plays a role in reducing the generation of free radicals in different tissues, including the brain. Numerous laboratory studies have indicated that animals with magnesium deficiency are more susceptible to oxidative stress.[216]

Magnesium supplementation has shown notable benefits in alleviating symptoms of daily psychological stress and anxiety, including fatigue, irritability, and sleep disturbances. Research suggests that individuals experiencing mental and physical stress and/or anxiety may benefit from regular magnesium intake. In a study looking at male students under common stressors like sleep deprivation, mild anxiety, lack of movement and poor nutrition, receiving 250 mg/day of magnesium for four weeks, not only exhibited increased erythrocyte magnesium levels but also reduced interleukin-6 (a marker of inflammation) and serum cortisol levels.[392] Moreover, supplementation with 400 mg/day of magnesium was linked to improved heart rate variability, indicating a more robust response to stress in subjects engaged in moderate muscle endurance training.[393] Heart rate variability is often used as a gauge of how the parasympathetic and vagal nervous systems respond to stress.[394] Daily supplementation with 300 mg of magnesium, with or without vitamin B6, led to stress relief, particularly in individuals reporting high stress levels at baseline, with significant reductions in Depression and Anxiety Stress Scale scores.[395] It is also important to note that low magnesium levels can lead to pyridoxine (vitamin B6) deficiency, affecting serotonin levels linked to depression, anxiety, and pain perception. Additionally, Vitamin B6 facilitates magnesium entry into cells and is also required for its intracellular buildup.[144, 395]

Magnesium deficiency, anxiety and stress are prevalent in the general population and can pose long-term health risks. While severe magnesium deficiency is uncommon, chronic latent deficiency is widespread, especially among individuals with anxiety and stress disorders.[1] While current dietary magnesium intake may prevent obvious signs of deficiency in most people, it might not be enough to promote optimal health and reduce the risk of chronic disease that can be triggered by persistent stress and anxiety.

Depression

Depression is a complex mental health condition that affects millions of people worldwide. It is characterized by persistent feelings of sadness, hopelessness, and a loss of interest in activities once enjoyed. Alongside these emotional symptoms, individuals may experience changes in appetite or weight, sleep disturbances, fatigue, difficulty concentrating, and thoughts of self-harm or suicide.[396] Depression can have a profound impact on various aspects of life, including work, relationships, and overall well-being, leading to a diminished quality of life.[396] Statistics indicate that about 3.8% of the population, including 5% of adults and 5.7% of the elderly, grapple with depression, underscoring its prevalence and potential impact on various age groups.[397] While treatment options such as psychotherapy and medications are effective in improving the symptoms of depression; over half of the patients who utilized medications reported experiencing side effects.[398] Studies have shown a potential role for magnesium in managing depressive symptoms, with minimal side effects. Understanding the connection between magnesium levels and depression may offer novel avenues for intervention and improved mental health outcomes.

Magnesium serves as a vital co-factor for a multitude of enzymes in the human body, many of which are crucial for brain function. It plays a role in mood regulation by maintaining the balance of key chemical compounds in the brain.[343] Magnesium also boosts the expression of brain-derived neurotrophic factor, which helps regulate the activity of the N-methyl-D-aspartic acid receptor.[399] Brain-derived neurotrophic factor is a protein found in the brain and peripheral nervous system that plays a crucial role in promoting the survival, growth, and maintenance of neurons.[400] It is important for synaptic plasticity, which is the ability of synapses (connections between neurons) to strengthen or weaken over time in response to activity. This protein is involved in various cognitive functions such as learning, memory, and mood regulation.[400] Changes in brain-derived neurotrophic factor levels have been linked to several neurological and psychiatric disorders, including depression, Alzheimer's disease, and schizophrenia.[401] By acting as an antagonist to the N-methyl-D-aspartic acid receptor complex and inhibiting glycogen synthase kinase 3 (GSK-3), magnesium exhibits effects similar to those of commonly used antidepressants.[399]

The exact mechanisms underlying the antidepressant effects of magnesium are not yet fully understood, but it likely affects various systems linked to depression.[402] Magnesium acts as a natural antagonist to calcium, blocking the N-methyl-D-aspartic acid receptor channel and preventing the flow of calcium ions through it. Additionally, magnesium enhances the expression of the GluN2B subunit of the N-methyl-D-aspartic acid receptor complex, which helps modulate glutamate neurotransmission implicated in mood regulation.[399] Low magnesium levels in the hippocampus, combined with high levels of calcium and glutamate, may disrupt synaptic functioning in the brain, leading to mood disorders such as depression.[403] Moreover, magnesium intake has been linked to reduced systemic inflammation, a significant risk factor for psychological disorders.[404] Early reports dating back almost one hundred years ago suggested the beneficial effects of magnesium sulfate in treating agitated depression. Subsequent pre-clinical and clinical studies have supported these findings and highlighted the safety of magnesium supplementation.[402] Consequently, magnesium supplementation appears to be well tolerated and can improve the effectiveness of conventional antidepressant therapies.[402]

Common conventional medications for depression are selective serotonin reuptake inhibitors. These medications work by increasing the levels of serotonin, a neurotransmitter in the brain associated with mood regulation, by blocking its reabsorption into the nerve cells.[405] Research has shown that magnesium's antidepressant effects seem to also involve modulation of the serotonin system.[406] When administered with selective serotonin reuptake inhibitors, magnesium shows a synergistic effect. Conversely, inhibiting serotonin synthesis impairs magnesium's antidepressant action.[406]

Given the prevalence of magnesium deficiency in the population, it is imperative to explore its role in contributing to depression and mood disorders. Studies have shown that magnesium deficiency contributes to mood disorders.[402] Recent research on depression has revealed a connection between the onset of this debilitating condition and diminished levels of magnesium in the bloodstream, a finding that is consistent with prior meta-analyses. It has been proposed that adults seen in primary care facilities with lower serum magnesium levels tend to exhibit depressive symptoms, thereby advocating for the use of magnesium supplementation as a therapeutic approach.[407-409] It has also been theorized that low magnesium levels might be a secondary biochemical characteristic in depressed patients who are less responsive to medication. Additionally, it's possible that individuals with lower magnesium levels and heightened activity traits represent a distinct biological subgroup with increased catecholaminergic activity and a limited response to certain antidepressant medications.[410] Furthermore, magnesium depletion may contribute to the link between low magnesium levels and unfavorable treatment outcomes, prompting investigation into the therapeutic potential of magnesium in depression.[410]

Patients experiencing treatment-resistant depression demonstrate reduced levels of magnesium in the central nervous system compared to healthy individuals. To address this, incorporating magnesium supplementation alongside standard antidepressant therapy may enhance treatment outcomes for depressed individuals with low magnesium levels, offering a personalized approach to managing depression.[410] In a 2008 clinical trial, magnesium was found to be as effective as the antidepressant Imipramine in treating depression in diabetic patients but without the associated side effects.[411] It was hypothesized that inadequate dietary magnesium could be the primary cause of treatment resistant depression, and physicians should consider prescribing magnesium for this condition.[411] Low brain magnesium levels are associated with reduced serotonin levels and antidepressants have been shown to have the action of raising brain magnesium. Thus, magnesium treatment may benefit not only treatment resistant depression but also other forms of depression.[412]

Postpartum depression is a significant form of depression typically occurring within 6 to 12 weeks after childbirth, although it can manifest up to a year later. In developed nations, the prevalence of postnatal depression ranges from 6-20% in adult women, varying based on diagnostic criteria and screening methods.[413] Mothers experiencing depressive symptoms often exhibit more complicated interactions with their children, potentially straining family bonds and, in extreme cases, leading to instances of infanticide.[414] As we have mentioned, magnesium plays a crucial role in the nervous system, affecting the release and metabolism of neurotransmitters. During pregnancy, significant amounts of nutrients, including magnesium, are absorbed by the fetus and placenta from the mother. This depletion of magnesium, coupled with insufficient intake by the mother, is theorized to contribute to postpartum depression. Additionally, lactation further depletes maternal magnesium levels.[414]

Understanding depression involves exploring various factors beyond just brain chemistry, and recent studies have revealed the crucial influence of the gut microbiome on mental health. The complex interplay between the gut and the brain, known as the gut-brain axis, has emerged as a key player in mood regulation, suggesting that the composition of our gut bacteria may play a significant role in the development and management of depression.[415] Previous research has linked changes in rodent behavior to alterations in the gut microbiota, which can be influenced by diet composition. Studies have demonstrated that a magnesium-deficient diet can lead to anxiety and depressive-like behavior in both humans and rodents. This suggests that the disruptions in the microbiota-gut-brain axis caused by a magnesium-deficient diet may contribute to the onset of depressive-like symptoms.[415]

A recent systematic review and meta-analysis demonstrated a notable impact of magnesium supplementation on reducing depression symptoms across various assessment tools.[397] Consistent with many findings, the effectiveness of magnesium in alleviating depression was well supported. Additionally, a study by Afsharfar et al. found that daily administration of 500 mg of magnesium for eight weeks can improve depression outcomes in adults.[416] Tarleton et al. found that a 2-week intervention with 248 mg of elemental magnesium daily improved clinical outcomes in individuals with anxiety and depressive disorders.[417] It is theorized that magnesium therapy could effectively treat major depression associated with intraneuronal magnesium deficiencies. These deficits may stem from stress hormones, excessive dietary calcium, or magnesium deficiencies.[418] Case studies demonstrate swift improvement (within 7 days) from major depression with the use of 125-300 mg of magnesium (as glycinate and taurinate) taken with meals and before bedtime.[418] Epidemiological and observational studies have shown a connection between higher dietary magnesium intake and a decreased risk of depressive disorders or fewer symptoms of depression.[419, 420]

Systemic inflammation, linked to decreased magnesium intake and depression, prompts exploration into magnesium's role in depressive disorders. Jacka et. al. investigated the connection between magnesium intake and depression/anxiety in a large community-based sample from Western Norway. The sample consisted of 5708 individuals aged 46-49 or 70-74 years. Results showed a negative correlation between magnesium intake and depression scores, unaffected by age, gender, or body measures.[421] Even after adjusting for socioeconomic and lifestyle factors, this association remained significant. Magnesium intake was also associated with reduced odds of depression cases.[421] It is important to note that magnesium intake could play an important role in supporting depression within communities, offering potential implications for public health and treatment strategies.

In a study from Tarleton et al. medical records from 3604 adults were analyzed in primary care clinics.[409] They found a significant relationship between serum magnesium levels and depression scores measured by the Patient Health Questionnaire (a measure of depression scores). Even after accounting for factors like age, gender, and health conditions, lower serum magnesium levels were consistently associated with higher depression scores.[409] These findings suggest that magnesium supplementation could be beneficial for adults experiencing depressive symptoms, and serum magnesium levels may help identify those who could benefit most from supplementation.

As depression continues to be a growing concern with substantial societal implications, exploring effective treatment options is paramount. Further research elucidating the mechanisms of magnesium's antidepressant effects and optimizing its clinical application will be crucial. Nevertheless, the growing body of evidence thus far highlights magnesium as a valuable adjunctive therapy in the comprehensive management of depression, offering hope and relief to those affected by this pervasive disorder.

Bipolar Disorder

Bipolar disorder, encompassing both Bipolar I and Bipolar II classifications, presents a formidable challenge to individuals and society alike. This mental health condition is marked by extreme mood swings between highs (mania or hypomania) and lows (depression), which can profoundly impact quality of life.[422] Bipolar I disorder involves episodes of severe mania, often requiring hospitalization, interspersed with periods of major depression.[422] In contrast, Bipolar II disorder is characterized by hypomanic episodes that are less severe than full-blown mania but still disruptive, alternating with depressive episodes.[422]

The economic burden of bipolar disorder is substantial, stemming from healthcare utilization, lost productivity, and social welfare support.[423] Conventional treatments typically involve mood-stabilizing medications like lithium or anticonvulsants, along with psychotherapy and lifestyle adjustments. However, many individuals experience inadequate symptom control, side effects, or resistance to medications.[423]

Given these challenges, there is growing interest in complementary approaches to bipolar disorder management. Magnesium, a crucial mineral involved in various bodily processes, has emerged as a potential adjunctive therapy. By modulating neurotransmitter activity, reducing inflammation, and promoting neuroplasticity, magnesium supplementation offers promise in enhancing mood stability and reducing symptom severity.[344] Exploring the efficacy of magnesium in conjunction with conventional treatments could provide a valuable avenue for improving outcomes in individuals with bipolar disorder, addressing a pressing need for effective interventions in mental health care.

Magnesium plays a crucial role in bipolar disorder by influencing both excitatory and inhibitory systems in the central nervous system. Low magnesium levels have been linked to reduced GABA activity (inhibitory in nature) in the neocortex and heightened response to glutamate (excitatory in nature) through N-methyl-D-aspartate receptor activation.[424] In patients with bipolar disorder, the levels of the serotonin transporter are lower by 16-26% in certain brain regions like the hypothalamus and amygdala compared to those without the disorder.[425-427] Studies on mice have shown that inhibiting serotonin synthesis or blocking 5-HT1 receptors diminishes the antidepressant-like effects of magnesium.[406] Magnesium has also been found to reduce serotonin turnover in animal brains exposed to stress. Additionally, magnesium's antidepressant effects were enhanced when combined with sub-effective doses of fluoxetine or imipramine, both of which are antidepressants.[406] In summary, serotonin promotes the release of GABA in certain brain areas, and magnesium, by increasing serotonin levels, can boost GABA release, thus helping to restore the disrupted balance between glutamate and GABA actions in mood disorders.

Research also shows that chronic magnesium deficiency is associated with higher rates of insulin resistance, type II diabetes mellitus, and depression.[428] Both major depression and depressive episodes in bipolar disorder patients show increased insulin resistance.[429] Supplementation with magnesium has been shown to alleviate both insulin resistance and depression.[417] While the exact biochemical link between insulin resistance and depression remains unclear, factors such as increased glutamate, reduced brain-derived neurotrophic factor (plays an important role in neuronal survival and growth), and peroxisome proliferator-activated receptor gamma[430] (causes insulin sensitization and enhances glucose metabolism[431]) are thought to play a role. Studies have shown that magnesium acts by blocking the calcium channel linked to N-methyl-D-aspartate receptors, thereby decreasing the release of glutamate in the brain.[432] Supplementation with magnesium for a duration of six weeks resulted in increased expression of peroxisome proliferator-activated receptor gamma and glucose transporter-1 genes (helps in the transport of glucose[433]). Additionally, reduced activity of sodium-potassium ATPase in bipolar disorder leads to decreased neuronal ion exchange, resulting in lower intraneuronal magnesium levels and higher intracellular calcium levels.[434]

The concentration of magnesium in the cerebrospinal fluid among individuals with mood disorders remains underexplored. Studies have revealed an elevated calcium/magnesium ratio in both cerebrospinal fluid and serum among those with major depression and individuals experiencing depressive episodes in bipolar disorder.[435] This heightened ratio has also been associated with manic agitation.[436] Additionally, research has indicated lower cerebrospinal fluid magnesium levels in individuals with a history of suicide attempts during depressive states compared to normal controls.[437]

Elevated oxidative stress plays a role in both bipolar disorder and major depression.[438] Patients with these conditions have lower levels of glutathione in their brains and higher levels of free radicals leading to mitochondrial damage. Additionally, individuals experiencing acute depressive episodes show reduced total antioxidant capacity.[439] To address this, reducing oxidative stress is considered a potential treatment approach.

Magnesium is known for its antioxidant and anti-inflammatory properties, suppressing the synthesis of proinflammatory cytokines and reducing oxidative stress.[364]

Numerous studies have indicated elevated levels of cortisol and adrenocorticotropic hormone in individuals with bipolar disorder, both during manic and depressive phases.[440] Compared to those with major depression and healthy controls, bipolar disorder patients consistently exhibit higher cortisol levels. Additionally, adrenocorticotropic hormone levels, both basal and peak concentrations, are elevated in bipolar disorder patients.[441] Hypomagnesemia, or decreased magnesium levels in the blood, contributes to hypothalamic-pituitary adrenal axis dysfunction, leading to increased synthesis of adrenocorticotropic hormone and cortisol.[384] Magnesium plays a modulatory role in this axis, reducing the secretion of adrenocorticotropic hormone and cortisol, thereby potentially alleviating symptoms associated with bipolar disorder.[384]

In conclusion, despite some of the variability in clinical study results, existing data consistently supports the therapeutic potential of magnesium in bipolar disorder. However, further research is warranted to elucidate the optimal timing, duration, and dosages of magnesium administration for maximizing its efficacy as a treatment in bipolar disorders. Moving forward, additional clinical studies can help to refine the use of magnesium as an adjunctive therapy in the management of bipolar disorder.

Schizophrenia Disorder

Schizophrenia is a chronic and severe mental disorder, posing significant challenges to individuals, families, and societies worldwide. Characterized by disruptions in thought processes, perceptions, and emotions, schizophrenia profoundly impacts an individual's ability to function in daily life. This disorder often emerges in late adolescence or early adulthood and persists throughout a person's lifetime, leading to considerable morbidity and mortality.[442]

Beyond its individual burden, schizophrenia also exacts a heavy toll on society, both economically and socially. The societal costs associated with schizophrenia are staggering, encompassing healthcare expenses, loss of productivity, and the strain on caregivers and support systems. Moreover, individuals with schizophrenia experience heightened rates of unemployment, homelessness, and incarceration, further underscoring the profound societal implications of this disorder.[442]

In addition to its socioeconomic impact, schizophrenia is associated with increased morbidity and mortality rates, largely attributable to comorbid physical health conditions, such as cardiovascular disease, diabetes, and respiratory illnesses. Furthermore, individuals with schizophrenia face heightened risks of self-harm, suicide, and premature death, highlighting the urgent need for effective interventions and treatments.[442]

In recent years, researchers have explored alternative approaches to managing schizophrenia, including the potential role of magnesium supplementation. Magnesium has garnered attention for its neuroprotective properties and its potential to modulate brain function.[426] Preliminary studies suggest that magnesium may offer a safe and effective adjunctive treatment for schizophrenia, prompting further investigation into its therapeutic potential and mechanisms of action.

Recognizing magnesium's critical role as a cofactor in the metabolism of various vitamins and neurotransmitters, and its potential implications for schizophrenia, a study conducted by J.D. Kanofsky and R. Sandykto assessed serum magnesium levels in a cohort of chronic institutionalized schizophrenic patients.[443] Among the 20 patients, 25% exhibited low serum magnesium levels ranging from 1.4 to 1.7 mg/dl, falling below the normal range of 1.8 to 2.4 mg/dl. Notably, none of the patients displayed abnormalities in other electrolyte levels, including sodium, potassium, chloride, calcium, and phosphorus. Interestingly, one patient demonstrated a significant reduction in psychotic symptoms after oral magnesium supplementation. They also observed that magnesium levels did not normalize with oral supplementation. This suggests the possibility of an absorption disturbance in a subset of patients, or the deficiency of magnesium was severe, potentially requiring higher supplementation doses.[443]

The clinical significance of magnesium deficiency in schizophrenia is underscored by its potential to disrupt the metabolism of essential nutrients such as thiamine (Vitamin B1), pyridoxine (Vitamin B6), vitamin E, vitamin C, zinc, copper, and selenium.[444] For example, magnesium deficiency can lead to decreased tissue thiamine levels, affecting serotonin synthesis, and impair the metabolism of pyridoxine, which is crucial for serotonin and GABA synthesis. Additionally, hypomagnesemia may enhance central cholinergic activity due to its inhibitory effect on acetylcholine release, which aligns with biochemical markers of negative schizophrenia.[443] Another study hypothesized that severely ill psychiatric patients may experience marginal magnesium deficiency due to elevated stress levels. This deficiency could worsen symptoms like anxiety, fear, hallucinations, weakness, and physical complaints.[445]

In addition, magnesium's impact suggests a multifaceted mechanism for its effect. Magnesium can reduce neuronal reactions to glutamate on N-methyl-D-aspartate receptors, limit glutamate release, mitigate peroxide radical formation, and enhance GABAergic activity and glycine synthesis.[426] Glycine synthesis inhibits catecholamine release[446] (dopamine and norepinephrine), which is often elevated in schizophrenic patients.[447, 448]

Given the poor prognosis and treatment resistance often seen in schizophrenic patients, magnesium deficiency may exacerbate neuroleptic nonresponsiveness and contribute to chronic institutionalization. The study by J.D. Kanofsky and R. Sandykto concluded that it is important to advocate for routine assessment of serum magnesium levels in chronic schizophrenic patients, with efforts directed toward correcting underlying deficiencies.[443] Addressing magnesium deficiency may potentially alleviate psychotic symptoms and reduce sensitivity to neuroleptic-induced extrapyramidal symptoms, thereby offering a novel avenue for improving treatment outcomes in schizophrenia.[443]

Attention-deficit/hyperactivity disorder (ADHD)

Attention-deficit/hyperactivity disorder (ADHD) is a neurodevelopmental disorder characterized by persistent patterns of inattention, hyperactivity, and impulsivity that significantly impair daily functioning.[449] While often associated with children, ADHD can persist into adulthood, affecting individuals of all ages. Children with ADHD may struggle with maintaining attention in school, completing tasks, and following instructions, leading to academic underachievement and behavioral challenges. Adults with ADHD may face difficulties in managing responsibilities at work, maintaining relationships, and organizing daily tasks.[450]

The increasing rates of ADHD diagnosis raise concerns about overdiagnosis and overmedication, prompting debates about appropriate identification and management. This trend has significant societal implications, including the economic burden on families and society stemming from healthcare costs, educational support, and lost productivity.[449] Amidst ongoing research, there is growing interest in exploring the potential benefits of magnesium supplementation as a complementary approach to managing ADHD symptoms.

A deficiency in magnesium is associated with cognitive impairments, leading to symptoms such as fatigue, difficulty concentrating, nervousness, mood swings, and aggression.[451] Given that these symptoms are often present in ADHD, it's unsurprising that clinical trials consistently show lower serum magnesium levels in patients with ADHD compared to healthy individuals.[451] In a study that looked at the assessment of magnesium levels in children with ADHD, 95% percent of the examined children with ADHD were found to have magnesium deficiency.[452] The highest occurrence of magnesium deficiency was found in hair (77.6%), followed by red blood cells (58.6%) and blood serum (33.6%).[452]

Magnesium plays a crucial role in regulating various brain functions, including behavior, by affecting neurotransmitters like dopamine, norepinephrine, and serotonin. Magnesium engages with the noradrenergic and dopaminergic systems. These systems have been thoroughly investigated in the context of ADHD's underlying mechanisms.[453] Moreover, stimulants and atomoxetine used to treat those with ADHD function via adrenergic and dopaminergic receptors.[454] Additionally, magnesium inhibits the release of norepinephrine induced by n-methyl-d-aspartate.[455] Therefore, magnesium deficiency may be linked to ADHD's pathophysiology, suggesting that magnesium supplementation may be beneficial as a therapeutic option for treating ADHD.[455, 456] In a study conducted by Starobrat-Hermelin B. and Kozielec T., it was shown that children who underwent magnesium supplementation for a duration of six months exhibited an increase in magnesium levels in their hair.[457] Moreover, they experienced a significant decrease in hyperactivity, both in comparison to their baseline condition and to the control group that did not receive magnesium treatment.[457] These findings suggest that magnesium supplementation may effectively alleviate hyperactivity in children, regardless of any accompanying mental disorders.

The synergistic relationship between magnesium and vitamin B6 underscores their combined therapeutic potential, particularly in conditions like ADHD where neurotransmitter imbalance plays a significant role.[456] Vitamin B6 plays a crucial role in synthesizing numerous neurotransmitters, such as GABA, serotonin, dopamine, noradrenaline, histamine, glycine, and d-serine.[458] Another suggested mechanism is that vitamin B6 aids in the cellular absorption of magnesium, reducing its excretion and enhancing its efficacy, given that magnesium primarily functions as an intracellular cation.[395] In a study involving 40 children diagnosed with ADHD; they received a regimen of magnesium-vitamin B6 treatment for a duration of at least 8 weeks. Clinical symptoms of ADHD were assessed and included hyperactivity, emotional instability/aggressiveness, and lack of attention at school. They also took measurements of intra-erythrocyte magnesium and blood ionized calcium. The magnesium-vitamin B6 regimen led to significant improvements in ADHD symptoms, particularly in reducing hyperactivity and emotional instability/aggressiveness, and enhancing school attention. Additionally, intra-erythrocyte magnesium values increased significantly with the magnesium-vitamin B6 treatment. Interestingly, the symptoms reappeared upon discontinuation of treatment, accompanied by a decrease in intra-erythrocyte magnesium values.[459]

Research also indicates a connection between magnesium and vitamin D. A high intake of total, dietary or supplemental magnesium is independently associated with a significantly reduced risk of vitamin D deficiency and insufficiency, respectively.[460] This is because magnesium is a cofactor for the enzymes that make vitamin D.[461] In a study conducted by Hemamy, M et al., they found that administration of vitamin D and magnesium to children diagnosed with ADHD led to reductions in conduct issues, social challenges, and anxiety/shyness ratings compared to those who received a placebo.[462]

The findings from studies investigating magnesium supplementation in individuals with ADHD suggest promising outcomes, indicating its potential as a beneficial intervention. It's apparent that ensuring adequate magnesium intake, either through supplementation or dietary adjustments, could offer significant advantages for those with ADHD symptoms. Understanding the etiology and impact of low micronutrient status, particularly magnesium, is crucial given its fundamental role in neurotransmitter production associated with ADHD. This ongoing exploration holds promise for advancing our understanding and identifying therapeutic strategies to better support individuals with ADHD.

Neurological Disorders

Neurological disorders encompass a vast array of conditions affecting the brain, spinal cord, and nerves, presenting significant challenges to individuals, families, and society as a whole. From Alzheimer's disease to epilepsy, these disorders vary widely in their symptoms, severity, and impact on daily life.[463] Not only do they pose immense burdens on patients and their caregivers, but they also exact a heavy toll on society, both economically and socially. The cost of neurological disorders, in terms of healthcare expenditures, lost productivity, and diminished quality of life, is staggering, running into the billions annually.[464] Moreover, the morbidity and mortality associated with these disorders are profound, with many conditions leading to debilitating disabilities or even premature death. Globally, millions of people are affected by neurological disorders, with the numbers rising steadily due to aging populations and other demographic shifts.[464]

Amidst these challenges, there is growing interest in exploring alternative or adjunctive treatments for neurological disorders, and magnesium has emerged as a promising avenue of investigation. Research suggests that magnesium plays a vital role in various neurological functions, including neurotransmitter regulation, neuronal signaling, and neuroprotection.[344] Given its potential neuroprotective and neuromodulatory properties, there is increasing interest in understanding how magnesium supplementation or dietary adjustments may impact the development and progression of these neurological disorders.

Alzheimer's / Dementia

Alzheimer's disease and dementia represent two of the most prevalent and challenging neurodegenerative disorders of our time, characterized by progressive cognitive decline and memory loss.[465] Alzheimer's disease, the most common form of dementia, gradually erodes an individual's ability to think, reason, and perform daily tasks, ultimately robbing them of their independence and identity. Symptoms typically begin with mild forgetfulness and confusion, eventually escalating to profound memory loss, disorientation, language difficulties, and impaired judgment. As the disease advances, individuals may experience personality changes, agitation, and difficulty with motor functions.[465]

The consequences of Alzheimer's disease and dementia extends far beyond the individual affected, profoundly impacting families and caregivers.[466] The financial burden of these conditions is staggering, with billions spent annually on healthcare costs, long-term care, and lost productivity. Moreover, the emotional toll on caregivers can be overwhelming, leading to increased stress, depression, and decreased quality of life.[466]

In the United States alone, Alzheimer's disease affects millions of individuals, with the number expected to rise dramatically in the coming decades as the population ages. Currently, it is estimated that over 6 million Americans are living with Alzheimer's disease, and this number is projected to triple by 2050 if no significant advancements are made in prevention and treatment.[466]

Amidst these challenges, there is growing interest in exploring alternative and adjunctive treatments for Alzheimer's disease and dementia, and magnesium has emerged as a promising avenue of investigation. Research suggests that magnesium plays a crucial role in brain health, supporting neuronal function, reducing neuroinflammation, and promoting synaptic plasticity.[343] By addressing magnesium deficiency and optimizing levels through supplementation or dietary interventions, we may potentially mitigate the risk of developing Alzheimer's disease and dementia, or possibly even slow the progression of these conditions.

Magnesium deficiency is linked to Alzheimer's disease, with lower magnesium levels found in the brains of these patients.[467] Although it's possible that a dysfunction in the blood-brain barrier affects magnesium transport, the exact causes are still unclear. A recent analysis of 21 studies found that Alzheimer's patients have significantly lower circulating magnesium levels compared to healthy individuals.[468] Considering that

Western diets often lack magnesium[1], it's noteworthy that higher dietary magnesium intake is linked to a lower risk of cognitive impairment.[75] In a recent study done in 2023 they followed 6,000 participants aged 40 to 73, all free of neurological issues, and tracked them over 16 months.[469] Researchers identified a connection between dietary magnesium and increased brain volume, notably in gray and white matter, indicating a significant neuroprotective impact, particularly in the gray matter and hippocampus. Compared to those with a standard magnesium intake of around 350 mg per day, individuals consuming over 550 mg displayed brain aging approximately one year younger than their chronological age by age 55.[469] The lead researcher stressed that a 41% increase in magnesium intake (550mg per day) correlated with reduced age-related brain shrinkage as well as potentially enhancing cognitive function and a lower risk of or delayed onset of dementia in later life.[469] What was interesting to note is that the neuroprotective effects of magnesium reached statistical significance exclusively in women. Furthermore, the effect was more pronounced in post-menopausal women than in their pre-menopausal counterparts, potentially owing to magnesium's anti-inflammatory properties.[469]

In animal models of Alzheimer's disease, magnesium supplementation has shown promise in reducing neuroinflammation, preventing the buildup of harmful proteins (amyloid beta-protein), and enhancing learning and memory abilities.[470]

Impaired insulin signaling seems to heighten the likelihood of Alzheimer's onset. This association is notable enough for some to label Alzheimer's as "diabetes of the brain" or "type 3 diabetes".[471] Magnesium deficiency may partly explain the link between type 2 diabetes and Alzheimer's disease.[472] Magnesium deficiency leads to impaired glucose tolerance and insulin resistance.[473] This results in elevated insulin and blood sugar levels, which promote the accumulation of amyloid beta plaques and worsen neuroinflammation.[472, 474] Correcting magnesium levels could potentially address both conditions simultaneously.

Research has suggested that the protective effects of magnesium are attributed to its ability to decrease interleukin-1beta (IL-1β), a key inflammatory factor, thus inhibiting inflammation.[475] In a mouse model of Alzheimer's disease, magnesium L-threonate (which can elevate brain magnesium levels) reduced beta-amyloid plaques[470], which may be due to its ability to inhibit the enzyme responsible for initiating amyloid beta generation.[476] Additionally, it facilitates the removal of amyloid beta fibrils by regulating the blood-brain barrier's permeability and prevents the phosphorylation of tau protein.[470, 475] Insufficient magnesium levels elevate substance P, a neurotransmitter that heightens pain sensation, leading to compromised blood-brain barrier integrity and activation of glial cells (major mediators of neuroinflammation). This process triggers an upsurge in nitric oxide, prostaglandins, cytokines, calcium, and reactive oxygen species, eventually leading to neuroinflammation and neurodegeneration often seen in Alzheimer's and other neurodegenerative diseases.[343]

In Alzheimer's disease, there's evidence suggesting that glutamate release and uptake are disrupted, potentially leading to elevated levels of glutamate in the synaptic cleft. This excess glutamate triggers calcium influx into postsynaptic neurons via N-methyl-D-aspartate receptors, activating enzymes and free radicals, resulting in cell damage and neuron death.[477] Recent research has increasingly focused on the relationship between magnesium and N-methyl-D-aspartate receptors in neurodegenerative disorders. N-methyl-D-aspartate receptors play vital roles in various brain functions, including neuronal development and degeneration. These receptors are gated channels permeable to ions like calcium, sodium, and potassium, with magnesium blocking their activation. During learning and memory processes, glutamate release leads to depolarization of postsynaptic membranes, allowing calcium influx. Magnesium ions exit the N-methyl-D-aspartate receptors, permitting calcium influx, which facilitates memory formation and learning. Magnesium then closes the channels, halting calcium influx, signaling the end of stimulation.[344, 478] Excessive calcium influx can lead to neuronal excitotoxicity and cell damage, so magnesium's role in closing the channels helps maintain neuronal health and function.[343]

Promisingly, dietary supplementation with magnesium L-threonate surpasses other magnesium compounds like magnesium chloride, magnesium citrate, and magnesium gluconate in its ability to elevate magnesium levels in the brain.[479] Numerous studies have highlighted the positive impact of magnesium on treating degenerative conditions. Patients with dementia showed memory enhancement and symptom alleviation with nutritional magnesium supplementation.[480] Additionally, individuals with higher self-reported magnesium intake exhibited a reduced risk of developing dementia.[481] Thus, replenishing brain magnesium and improving magnesium deficiency could offer a promising avenue for addressing cognitive impairment in individuals with Alzheimer's disease. However, more studies are still needed to confirm the in-depth clinical application of magnesium.

Parkinson's Disease

Parkinson's disease is a progressive neurological disorder that is caused by degeneration of nerve cells in the part of the brain called the substantia nigra, which primarily affects movement. It occurs when nerve cells in the brain, particularly those responsible for producing dopamine, become damaged or die. Dopamine is a neurotransmitter involved in regulating movement and emotions. As Parkinson's disease progresses, individuals may experience tremors, stiffness, slowness of movement, and difficulty with balance and coordination. These symptoms can significantly impact daily life, making tasks such as walking, speaking, and completing simple actions challenging.[482]

Beyond its physical symptoms, Parkinson's disease also carries a significant burden on individuals and society. The disease can lead to decreased quality of life, increased disability, and a higher risk of complications such as falls and infections. Additionally, Parkinson's disease is associated with increased mortality rates, primarily due to complications related to immobility and the progression of the disease.[482]

Parkinson's disease has become the second most prevalent neurodegenerative disorder, experiencing a rapid increase in prevalence over the past two decades.[343] Given the complexity and impact of Parkinson's disease, there is a growing interest in exploring alternative and complementary approaches to its management. Magnesium has emerged as a potential candidate for intervention due to its role in neuronal function and neuroprotection. Research suggests that magnesium may play a protective role in neurodegenerative disorders by modulating neurotransmitter activity, reducing inflammation, and protecting against oxidative stress.[344]

Parkinson's disease arises from various pathological processes, including abnormal protein aggregation, lysosome dysfunction, mitochondrial dysfunction, endoplasmic stress, glutaminergic excitotoxicity, oxidative stress, and neuroinflammation.[483] These factors contribute to neuronal death, particularly affecting dopaminergic neurons

113

in the basal ganglia.[483] Magnesium may offer beneficial effects by counteracting oxidative stress, neuroinflammation, and excessive activity of N-methyl-D-aspartate receptors.[343] Additionally, magnesium increases brain-derived neurotrophic factor, which supports the health of dopaminergic neurons.[484] Moreover, magnesium regulates the mTOR pathway (essential cellular signaling pathway), reducing the formation of α-synuclein, a key protein implicated in Parkinson's disease pathology.[485]

Parkinson's patients have low magnesium concentrations in the cortex, white matter, basal ganglia, and brain stem.[486] It has also been shown that Parkinson's disease patients and animal models of the disease exhibit lower levels of magnesium in the cerebrospinal fluid compared to controls.[487] Animal studies have shown that prolonged low magnesium intake across generations can harm various cellular structures, including mitochondria, endoplasmic reticulum, ribosomes, and nuclear DNA, leading to the loss of dopaminergic neurons in the substantia nigra.[488] Interestingly, rats experiencing chronic low magnesium intake demonstrate a significant loss in dopaminergic neurons.[488]

Changes in heavy metal and mineral balance play a crucial role in neuronal functions, with disruptions in metal homeostasis linked to Parkinson's disease progression. Excessive levels of certain heavy metals/minerals like manganese, iron, lead, mercury, aluminum, and cadmium have been linked to damage in dopaminergic neurons, the cells primarily impacted in Parkinson's Disease.[489] However, magnesium is believed to act as a neuroprotective agent by inhibiting N-methyl-D-aspartate receptor activity and reducing oxidative stress.[490] Research indicates that insufficient magnesium levels may facilitate the accumulation of heavy metals in the brain, contributing to Parkinson's disease.[486, 491] According to one autopsy study, levels of calcium and aluminum were found to be elevated in the brains of individuals with Parkinson's compared to those with normal brain function.[486] It seems that these metals compete with magnesium for entry into brain cells. When magnesium levels are low, heavy metals can enter the cells more easily.[492]

In a mouse study, researchers utilized magnesium-L-threonate, a magnesium compound known for its ability to penetrate the blood-brain barrier effectively.[493] The findings

114

revealed that magnesium-L-threonate, unlike magnesium sulfate, elevated the magnesium level in the cerebrospinal fluid. These results suggest that the beneficial effects of magnesium L-threonate may be linked to the increased magnesium concentration in the cerebrospinal fluid following treatment. Notably, the cerebrospinal fluid magnesium concentration rose by approximately 21.6% after magnesium L-threonate treatment on day 28.[493] Furthermore, magnesium L-threonate demonstrated a notable ability to mitigate 1-methyl-4-phenyl-1,2,3,6-tetrahydropyridine (MPTP)-induced motor deficits and dopamine neuronal degeneration in mice, in contrast to magnesium sulfate. MPTP is a chemical that can lead to Parkinson's-like symptoms by harming certain neurons in the brain. It's often used in research to create models of Parkinson's disease in animals.[494]

Human studies on magnesium levels in Parkinson's disease are notably scarce, despite emerging evidence from animal research suggesting its importance. More studies are required in Parkinson's patients to establish a clearer understanding of the connection between magnesium and the disease.

Amyotrophic Lateral Sclerosis (ALS)

Amyotrophic Lateral Sclerosis (ALS), often referred to as Lou Gehrig's disease, is a progressive and devastating neurodegenerative disorder that affects the nerve cells in the brain and spinal cord. This debilitating condition leads to the gradual loss of voluntary muscle movement, eventually resulting in paralysis. ALS not only impacts physical abilities but also affects speech, swallowing, and eventually, breathing.[495]

The mortality rate of ALS is high, with most individuals succumbing to respiratory failure within three to five years of diagnosis. Furthermore, the disease imposes significant morbidity, greatly diminishing the quality of life for those affected and placing immense emotional and financial burdens on patients and their families.[495] As researchers strive to uncover effective treatments and ultimately a cure for ALS, the urgent need for greater awareness and support for those living with this challenging condition remains paramount.

Deficiencies in calcium and magnesium have been linked to neuropathology.[344] Research has shown that monkeys on a low-calcium diet displayed brain changes similar

115

to early stages of ALS and Parkinson's disease.[496] Similarly, individuals with these conditions in certain populations were found to have low calcium levels. ALS patients also had lower magnesium levels compared to healthy individuals.[496] Prolonged low calcium exposure might disrupt the balance of calcium-dependent processes in cells, potentially affecting cell function and leading to cell death. Magnesium, crucial for metabolic processes, could also be harmful if deficient, especially in active cells like neurons.[496]

In a study by Yasui, M. et al. they looked at regions with a high incidence of ALS, like the Western Pacific. Dietary deficiencies in calcium and magnesium, coupled with excess intake of aluminum and manganese, are thought to contribute to the disease's development. Using neutron activation analysis, they measured aluminum, calcium, and phosphorus levels, while magnesium levels were determined using inductively coupled plasma emission spectrometry (ICP), across 26 central nervous system regions in six ALS cases and five neurologically normal controls. The ALS patients showed significantly elevated aluminum concentrations in specific central nervous system regions compared to controls. Conversely, magnesium concentrations were notably reduced in ALS cases, leading to increased calcium/magnesium ratios. These findings suggest that the high incidence of ALS in the Western Pacific may stem from disruptions in calcium and magnesium metabolism, resulting in aluminum deposition in the central nervous system.[497]

Unfortunately, scientific research on the relationship between ALS and magnesium is currently limited beyond the findings mentioned above. While these studies provide valuable insights into potential links between ALS and disturbances in calcium-magnesium metabolism, further research is needed to fully understand the role of magnesium in the development and progression of ALS. Future studies exploring magnesium's effects on ALS pathogenesis, its potential as a therapeutic intervention, and its interaction with other factors implicated in the disease could provide critical advancements in our understanding and management of ALS.

Traumatic Brain Injury

Traumatic brain injury is a significant public health concern characterized by damage to the brain caused by an external force. This force could result from various incidents, including falls, vehicle accidents, sports injuries, or assaults. Traumatic brain injury can lead to a wide range of physical, cognitive, emotional, and behavioral impairments, depending on the severity and location of the injury. Symptoms may include headaches, confusion, memory problems, difficulty concentrating, mood swings, and even coma in severe cases. The impact of a traumatic brain injury extends beyond individual suffering, with significant societal costs, including long-term disability and reduced quality of life for affected individuals.[498]

In recent years, there has been growing interest in the potential role of magnesium as a therapeutic intervention for traumatic brain injury, given its neuroprotective properties and potential to mitigate injury severity and improve outcomes. Indeed, magnesium is crucial for maintaining balance in the pathways implicated in the secondary phase of brain injury.[499] Primary injury is irreversible and occurs at the time of impact. Unlike primary injury, secondary injury is potentially reversible, thereby providing a therapeutic window for pharmacological intervention to reduce injury and improve both outcome and survival.[500] In cases of traumatic brain injury, decreased magnesium levels in the brain coincide with an influx of glutamate and calcium into the postsynaptic neuron. This influx is believed to be a primary driver of neuronal degeneration and cell death following the initial injury.[501] Additionally, magnesium's impact on the functioning of monoaminergic and serotonergic neurotransmitter systems suggests potential antidepressant effects in experimental studies. This is particularly relevant as disruptions in these systems are part of the secondary injury cascade after a traumatic brain injury.[502]

Excessive calcium influx into cells is considered a primary factor in brain damage, leading to heightened levels of free radicals, proteolysis (breakdown of proteins), apoptosis initiation, and inflammation.[503] Magnesium, a crucial ion in the central nervous system, plays vital roles in various physiological processes, including ischemia response, cellular energy metabolism, and protein synthesis. Acting as a potent calcium channel blocker, magnesium regulates intracellular calcium levels, thereby exerting protective effects.[503] Additionally, magnesium enhances cardiac output and cerebral blood flow. Deficient magnesium levels can elevate intracellular calcium, posing a risk in head injuries and correlating with poor neurological outcomes and increased mortality rates.[503] Replenishing magnesium levels may mitigate edema, enhance neurological and cognitive recovery, and alleviate ischemia-related issues.[503]

In a small study involving 30 patients with traumatic brain injury, supplementation with magnesium resulted in improved patient outcomes, as assessed by the Glasgow Coma Scale. [504] The Glasgow Coma Scale serves as the primary scoring system utilized to assess an individual's level of consciousness after experiencing a traumatic brain injury. Essentially, it aids in determining the severity of the injury.[505]

In situations of low magnesium levels, as seen after traumatic brain injury, immune cells experience heightened intracellular calcium, intensifying their reactivity.[506] This leads to a pronounced inflammatory reaction characterized by the activation of neurons, glia, and the infiltration of immune cells into the brain. Consequently, elevated levels of inflammatory cytokines such as interleukin (IL)-1B, IL-1, IL-6, and tumor necrosis factor alpha (TNF-a) were observed in both clinical patients and experimental models of trauma.[507, 508] These cytokines play pivotal roles in propagating the inflammatory cascade, promoting the release of damaging molecules like prostaglandins, reactive oxygen species, and proteases, ultimately contributing to blood-brain barrier dysfunction and the formation of cerebral edema.[500]

It is now widely accepted that a decrease in intracellular magnesium is a common occurrence in acute brain injury, with well-documented negative impacts on injury pathways and outcomes. Moreover, restoring magnesium levels in injured tissue to normal physiological levels is known to provide neuroprotection.[500]

Multiple Sclerosis

Multiple sclerosis is a chronic autoimmune disease that affects the central nervous system, including the brain and spinal cord. It is characterized by inflammation, demyelination (damage to the protective covering of nerve fibers), and the formation of scar tissue.[509] This results in a wide range of symptoms that can vary greatly among individuals, including fatigue, weakness, numbness or tingling in the limbs, difficulty with coordination and balance, vision problems, and cognitive impairment. Multiple sclerosis can significantly impact a person's quality of life, leading to disability and limitations in daily activities.[510]

While multiple sclerosis is not typically considered fatal, it can lead to complications that may shorten life expectancy. However, the course of multiple sclerosis varies widely among individuals, with some experiencing relatively mild symptoms and others facing more severe disability.[510] Currently, there is limited research on the relationship between magnesium and multiple sclerosis. However, the research that is available suggests that magnesium may play a beneficial role in managing multiple sclerosis symptoms and potentially slowing disease progression.

As mentioned, multiple sclerosis is characterized by demyelination and axonal degeneration in the brain and spinal cord, along with disruption of the blood-brain barrier, all driven by inflammation.[509] Cytokines, nitric oxide, and mitochondrial dysfunction play crucial roles in the disease's onset, recurrence, and progression. Given magnesium's anti-inflammatory properties and its role in mitochondrial function, it may offer protection against these mechanisms.[353, 509] Given that reduced magnesium levels trigger NF-kB activation (dysregulation of NF-κB activity can lead to chronic inflammation and contribute to the development of various diseases), the correlation between magnesium deficiency and heightened pro-inflammatory cytokine levels comes as no surprise.[343] Magnesium levels have been found to be reduced in the central nervous system tissues of individuals with multiple sclerosis, particularly in areas like white matter where pathological alterations are evident.[511]

It has been shown that vitamin D deficiency appears to contribute to the development of the disease, so it is important to highlight that magnesium is essential for the activation of vitamin D.[512] Therefore, magnesium supplementation is advised in cases of vitamin D deficiency.[513] Treatment with magnesium, calcium and vitamin D may reduce multiple sclerosis exacerbations.[514]

In conclusion, while the current body of research on magnesium and its effects on multiple sclerosis is modest, it holds promise for potential therapeutic applications. It is hoped that further investigation in this area will yield valuable insights that can positively impact the lives of individuals living with multiple sclerosis.

Epilepsy

Epilepsy is a neurological disorder characterized by recurrent seizures, which are sudden bursts of electrical activity in the brain. These seizures can vary widely in severity and manifestation, ranging from brief lapses of attention or muscle jerks to severe and prolonged convulsions.[515] Epilepsy affects approximately 50 million people globally and of all ages, from infants to the elderly.[344] This condition significantly impacts the quality of life of these individuals. This can result in various challenges, including restrictions on activities, limitations in employment opportunities, and social stigma. Moreover, epilepsy is associated with an increased risk of morbidity and mortality, particularly due to accidents, injuries during seizures, and complications from anti-seizure medications.[515]

Despite conventional treatments with anti-epileptic drugs, newer options have not significantly improved outcomes. This has spurred interest in alternative therapies like magnesium, given its potential neuroprotective and anti-seizure properties. [431]

Research has shown that excessive glutamatergic neurotransmission is closely associated with seizure activity. It has been suggested that magnesium may regulate excitotoxicity in epilepsy.[516] Studies indicate that extracellular magnesium can decrease spontaneous seizure spikes by acting on the N-methyl-D-aspartate receptor and reducing neuronal hyperexcitability. Hypomagnesemia, characterized by low magnesium levels, can itself trigger seizure activity, particularly in cases of severe deficiency.[517]

In humans, a deficiency in magnesium has been linked to seizures, and epileptic patients often exhibit lower magnesium levels compared to healthy individuals.[518, 519] A recent meta-analysis of 60 studies, including those on epilepsy and febrile seizures, showed no significant differences in magnesium levels between patients and controls. However, hair magnesium concentrations were notably lower in both untreated and treated epilepsy patients compared to controls.[520] Additionally, another study noted lower magnesium levels in more severe epilepsy cases and status epilepticus compared to milder cases.[521] Further exploration of the relationship between disease severity and magnesium concentration could yield valuable insights into epilepsy management.

Magnesium supplementation has proven beneficial in treating hypomagnesemia, a recognized seizure risk factor in both infants and adults. Moreover, conditions linked to symptomatic seizures, like pre-eclampsia and eclampsia, have shown improvement with magnesium supplementation.[344]

Although various research studies support the efficacy of magnesium treatment for epilepsy, only one randomized controlled trial has specifically investigated its use in infantile spasms. This study combined intravenous administration of adrenocorticotropic hormone with magnesium supplementation over three weeks, resulting in a significant reduction in seizures compared to the adrenocorticotropic hormone group alone. Eight weeks post-administration, the magnesium supplementation group exhibited a 79% seizure-free rate, whereas the adrenocorticotropic hormone only group showed only a 53% seizure-free rate.[522]

As a relatively safe and well-tolerated mineral, magnesium offers a potential adjunctive therapy for epilepsy alongside conventional anti-seizure medications. However, more randomized controlled trials are essential for gaining a deeper understanding of magnesium's potential as a treatment option for epilepsy. These trials would offer enhanced and targeted insights into magnesium's efficacy as a standalone or adjunct therapy for different forms of epilepsy.

Fibromyalgia

Fibromyalgia is a complex and debilitating disorder characterized by widespread musculoskeletal pain, fatigue, sleep disturbances, and cognitive difficulties. This chronic condition affects millions of individuals worldwide, predominantly women, although it can also occur in men and children.[523] Fibromyalgia significantly impacts daily functioning and quality of life, often leading to physical and emotional distress, social isolation, and impaired productivity. While fibromyalgia itself does not directly lead to mortality, its associated symptoms and complications can exacerbate existing health conditions and contribute to reduced life expectancy. Given the multifaceted nature of fibromyalgia and the limited effectiveness of conventional treatments, there is growing interest in exploring alternative therapies such as magnesium supplementation.

Fibromyalgia was initially considered a rheumatic disorder but is now known to be a neurological condition.[344, 524] The mechanism of pain transmission in fibromyalgia involves glutamate (the primary excitatory neurotransmitter in the brain) acting on the N-methyl-D-aspartate receptor.[523, 525] This suggests a potential protective role for magnesium in this condition. Fibromyalgia is hypothesized to stem from inadequate levels of essential substances crucial for adenosine triphosphate (ATP, the source of energy for use and storage at the cellular level) synthesis, including oxygen, magnesium, adenosine diphosphate (a molecule that is involved in transferring and providing cells with energy), and inorganic phosphate. Magnesium plays a vital role in this process since it is required for both aerobic and anaerobic glycolysis.[523] Furthermore, magnesium also assists in keeping cytosolic calcium levels low, thereby preventing the inhibition of adenosine triphosphate synthesis in the mitochondria, which helps decrease the risk of cell death due to mitochondrial calcification.[344]

Studies have found decreased levels of erythrocyte and intracellular muscle magnesium levels among fibromyalgia patients, while plasma and serum levels appear normal. However, other studies indicate significantly lower serum magnesium levels in fibromyalgia patients compared to controls.[344] A recent study investigated the effects of 300mg of magnesium citrate and 10mg of amitriptyline, alone and combined, in 60 women with fibromyalgia for eight weeks. Both erythrocyte and serum magnesium levels were lower in the fibromyalgia group. The combination of magnesium and amitriptyline resulted in reduced pain scores, while magnesium alone improved tender points and pain intensity.[524] Another study showed improved scores on the Fibromyalgia Impact Questionnaire-Revised after eight weeks of transdermal magnesium chloride solution use.[526]

In conclusion, the growing body of evidence points to magnesium as a promising treatment avenue for fibromyalgia. As research progresses and its mechanisms of action become clearer, magnesium supplementation could offer new hope for managing the symptoms and improving the well-being of those living with fibromyalgia.

Migraines

Migraines are prevalent neurological disorders characterized by intense, throbbing pain and discomfort.[527] While headaches are a common ailment experienced by many people at some point in their lives, migraines represent a more severe and debilitating form of headache, often accompanied by additional symptoms such as nausea, vomiting, and sensitivity to light and sound.[527] These conditions can significantly impair daily functioning and quality of life for affected individuals.

Migraines are estimated to affect around 1 billion people globally, making them one of the most prevalent neurological disorders worldwide. It is also worth mentioning that migraine is the second leading cause of disability worldwide.[528] The morbidity associated with migraines and headaches extends beyond the physical pain, impacting productivity, social interactions, and emotional well-being. While migraines and headaches are not typically associated with mortality, their chronic nature and severe symptoms can lead to significant long-term disability.[527] In addressing these conditions, magnesium has emerged as a promising treatment option due to its potential effectiveness and safety profile.

While the precise mechanisms are not fully understood yet, migraines are associated with changes in central nervous system excitability, spontaneous neuronal depolarization, and abnormal mitochondrial function.[529] Glutamate, a major excitatory neurotransmitter, is frequently implicated in discussions about migraine etiology, prevention, and treatment.[529] Magnesium has emerged as a potential treatment due to its ability to block the glutamatergic N-methyl-D-aspartate receptor, known for its role in pain transmission and cortical spreading depression.[530] Additionally, magnesium plays a crucial role in mitochondrial function and reduces membrane permeability, thus curbing hyperexcitability and spontaneous neuronal depression.[531]

The structure of the N-methyl-D-aspartate receptor, which is vital for glutamate release, is implicated in cortical depression initiation. Balanced magnesium and calcium levels are essential for N-methyl-D-aspartate receptor function, and disruptions in ion concentrations can affect cortical depression induction.[528] As mentioned, one of magnesium's key roles in the nervous system involves interacting with the N-methyl-D-aspartate receptor, where it blocks the calcium channel, guarding against excessive calcium entry into cells. Therefore, low magnesium levels can heighten glutamatergic neurotransmission, fostering excitotoxicity and ultimately triggering oxidative stress.[528] Neurological conditions like migraine, chronic pain, and epilepsy are thought to stem from abnormal glutamatergic neurotransmission.

Studies have reported significantly lower levels of magnesium in serum, saliva, and cerebrospinal fluid during and between migraine attacks[528], along with indications of reduced brain magnesium concentrations based on magnetic resonance spectroscopy (measures biochemical changes in the brain).[344] Trauninger et al. looked at whether individuals with migraines have a systemic deficiency of magnesium. An oral magnesium load test was performed by giving 3000 mg of magnesium lactate during a 24-hour period to 20 patients with migraine and 20 healthy controls. Despite serum and urine magnesium levels being similar, migraine patients retained significantly more magnesium after oral intake compared to healthy participants, indicating systemic magnesium deficiency.[532] A recent meta-analysis conducted by Chiu et al. in 2016 reviewed a broad array of randomized clinical trials, encompassing 11 studies on intravenous magnesium for acute migraines as well as 10 studies on oral magnesium for migraine prophylaxis.[533] The analysis utilized odds ratios (OR) to determine the effectiveness of magnesium treatment. Results showed that intravenous magnesium led to significant relief at 15-45 minutes (OR = 0.23), 120 minutes (OR = 0.20), and 24 hours (OR = 0.27) post-administration. Similarly, oral magnesium treatment significantly reduced the frequency (OR = 0.20) and intensity (OR = 0.27) of migraine attacks.[533] This meta-analysis highlights the efficacy of magnesium, whether administered intravenously or orally, in the treatment of migraines.

Dietary surveys in Western countries reveal magnesium intakes lower than the recommended dietary allowances, indicating widespread low magnesium intake.[1] This low intake is partly why magnesium deficiency is so common. As we have mentioned, to detect such deficiencies, sensitive tests assessing magnesium status are necessary. Due to magnesium being an intracellular cation, total or ionized magnesium levels in blood cells (such as lymphocytes or mononuclear blood cells, which are lymphocytes and monocytes) is recommended as the most suitable tests.[1, 175] In a study done by Thomas, J. et al. they measured total magnesium levels in plasma, erythrocytes, and lymphocytes in 29 migraine patients and 18 controls. Migraine patients exhibited significantly lower magnesium concentrations in erythrocytes and in lymphocytes compared to controls.[175] After a 2-week intake of magnesium-rich mineral water (containing 110 mg/L magnesium), there was a significant increase in all intracellular magnesium concentrations in migraine patients. There was no impact on plasma magnesium levels. This indicates good bioavailability of magnesium from this source. Magnesium in lymphocytes emerged as the most sensitive indicator of magnesium deficiency, showing a 15% decrease in migraine patients compared to controls, and a 16% increase after the mineral water intake.[175]

In a study involving various headache types, it was found that 42% of migraine patients had low serum ionized magnesium and a high ionized calcium to ionized magnesium ratio during an attack, compared to only 23% of patients with a severe continuous headache.[534] Reduced ionized magnesium levels and an elevated ionized calcium to ionized magnesium ratio could trigger cerebral vasospasm and diminish blood flow in the brain. Changes in ionized magnesium levels could also impact the function of serotonin receptors. Individuals with migraines who have low serum ionized magnesium levels or a high ionized calcium to ionized magnesium ratio might benefit from magnesium supplementation.[534] The recommended magnesium dosage according to the International, American, and European Headache Societies and the Neurological Academy ranges from 400 mg to 600 mg per day.[528, 535]

For almost two-thirds of women experiencing migraines, attacks coincide with their menstrual cycle. A menstrual migraine is typically identified as beginning between two days before a period and the third day of menstruation, often marked by heightened severity, longer duration, and increased sensitivity to light compared to non-menstrual migraines. The condition is attributed to a sudden decrease in estrogen levels preceding menstruation.[536] In a double-blind, placebo-controlled study, following a preliminary period of two menstrual cycles, the intervention began on the 15th day of the cycle. This consisted of either 360 mg/day of magnesium or placebo and persisted until the onset of the subsequent menstrual period, spanning two months. Subsequently, oral magnesium was administered in an open-label manner for the subsequent two months.[537] Magnesium treatment notably improved premenstrual complaints, evidenced by a significant decrease in Menstrual Distress Questionnaire (MDQ) scores. The number of days with a headache was also reduced. These improvements persisted at the fourth month of treatment when magnesium was supplemented in all patients.[537] It was shown that intracellular magnesium levels were reduced in patients with menstrual migraine compared to controls. During oral magnesium treatment, magnesium content in lymphocytes and polymorphonucleated cells significantly increased, while no changes were observed in plasma or red blood cells. An inverse correlation was noted between the Pain Total Index and magnesium content in polymorphonucleated cells.[537] These findings suggest that magnesium supplementation may be an additional approach for the prophylaxis of menstrual migraines. Furthermore, this indicates the potential association between magnesium deficiency and a decreased threshold for migraines.[537]

While current research highlights a strong role of magnesium in migraine management, further investigations are warranted. Maintaining adequate magnesium levels is essential for protecting neurons against excitotoxicity and oxidative stress[344], which may contribute to reducing migraine severity. Oral magnesium supplements emphasize their effectiveness and affordability by reducing migraine attack frequency and treatment costs. Thus, continued research into magnesium supplementation could offer promising avenues for improved migraine care and management.

Conclusion

In conclusion, the extensive and robust body of research surrounding magnesium and brain health underscores its profound impact on various aspects of neurological function. From aiding in the management of neurological disorders to promoting healthy sleep patterns and alleviating mood disorders, magnesium emerges as a powerful, safe, and effective nutrient for promoting overall brain well-being. Moreover, evidence consistently implicates magnesium deficiency in the onset and exacerbation of these conditions, emphasizing the critical importance of maintaining sufficient magnesium levels in the body.

As research in this field continues to evolve, it is evident that magnesium supplementation holds promise as a cornerstone in the management of sleep disturbances, mood imbalances, migraines, and other neurological disorders. With each new study, our understanding of magnesium's mechanisms of action and therapeutic potential deepens, paving the way for more targeted interventions and personalized treatment strategies. Therefore, it is imperative that individuals prioritize adequate magnesium intake through diet and supplementation to support optimal brain health and function. By remaining vigilant in our efforts to maintain adequate magnesium levels and staying attuned to emerging research findings, we can harness the full potential of this essential mineral to nurture a healthier brain and enhance overall well-being.

Chapter 5: Magnesium's Role in Insulin Resistance, Metabolic Syndrome, and Diabetes

Metabolic disorders are a group of conditions that disrupt the normal metabolic processes in the body. They often involve the intricate interplay between hormones and the metabolic pathways they regulate. Among these, insulin resistance, metabolic syndrome, and diabetes are particularly prominent due to their widespread prevalence and significant impact on health.[538] These disorders are not only medical concerns but also critical public health challenges, affecting millions of individuals worldwide and placing a substantial burden on healthcare systems.[539]

The prevalence of these metabolic endocrine disorders has been increasing globally, driven by rising obesity rates, sedentary lifestyles, and dietary changes.[540] According to the International Diabetes Federation, 10.5% of adults aged 20-79 have diabetes, with nearly half of them unaware of their condition. Projections by the International Diabetes Federation suggest that by 2045, approximately 783 million adults, or 1 in 8 globally, will be affected by diabetes, marking a 46% increase.[540] Insulin resistance and metabolic syndrome affect an even larger portion of the population, often serving as precursors to type 2 diabetes.[541]

These conditions have profound impacts on individual health and the healthcare system. They are associated with a range of complications, including cardiovascular disease, kidney failure, nerve damage, and vision problems. The chronic nature of these disorders requires ongoing medical management, which includes regular monitoring of blood glucose levels, medication adherence, lifestyle modifications, and sometimes, insulin therapy. This continuous care imposes a significant economic burden on healthcare systems, with diabetes alone accounting for a substantial portion of healthcare expenditures in many countries.[540]

Given the rising incidence of insulin resistance, metabolic syndrome, and diabetes, it is imperative to address these conditions through comprehensive public health strategies. This involves promoting healthier lifestyles, improving dietary habits, encouraging physical activity, and implementing preventive measures to reduce obesity. Early detection and management of these disorders are crucial in mitigating their progression and associated complications.

Emerging research suggests that magnesium plays a crucial role in the management and prevention of metabolic disorders. Studies have indicated that adequate magnesium intake is associated with a lower risk of developing insulin resistance, metabolic syndrome, and type 2 diabetes.[473] In short, magnesium's potential benefits include improving insulin sensitivity, reducing systemic inflammation, and enhancing glucose control.

In this chapter, we will dive deeper into insulin resistance, metabolic syndrome, and diabetes and explore the promising role of magnesium in mitigating these conditions. We will highlight its potential as an adjunctive treatment as well as a preventive measure. Addressing these disorders holistically is essential not only for improving individual health outcomes but also for alleviating the broader societal and economic impacts. As the prevalence of these metabolic disorders continues to rise, concerted efforts in research, public health, and clinical practice are paramount to curb their growing tide and enhance population health.

Insulin Resistance

Insulin resistance is a pathological condition in which the body's cells become less responsive to the hormone insulin. Insulin, produced by the pancreas, is critical for regulating blood glucose levels by facilitating the uptake of glucose into cells for energy production. When cells become resistant to insulin, the body compensates by producing more insulin, leading to a state of hyperinsulinemia. This condition can have significant repercussions on metabolic health and is a key precursor to type 2 diabetes and other serious health complications.

In a healthy individual, insulin binds to its receptor on the cell surface, triggering a series of intracellular events that allow glucose to enter the cell. In insulin resistance, these signaling pathways are impaired, often due to defects in the insulin receptor or downstream signaling molecules. This impairment reduces glucose uptake by muscle, fat, and liver cells, resulting in elevated blood glucose levels. Over time, the pancreas struggles to produce enough insulin to overcome this resistance, leading to progressively worsening hyperglycemia.[542]

The development of insulin resistance is multifactorial, with a combination of genetic, lifestyle, and environmental factors playing a role. Key contributors include obesity, a sedentary lifestyle, diets high in refined sugars and carbohydrates, genetics, and hormonal imbalances such as polycystic ovary syndrome (PCOS) and Cushing's syndrome.[542]

A recent analysis of the 2021 National Health and Nutrition Examination Survey data revealed that 40% of U.S. adults aged 18 to 44 exhibit insulin resistance according to HOMA-IR measurements.[543] Insulin resistance is alarmingly common and often goes undiagnosed because it can develop gradually and without obvious symptoms. However, its consequences are profound, significantly contributing to the global burden of chronic diseases. Insulin resistance is associated with the development of various diseases, such as cardiovascular disease, metabolic syndrome, obesity, cancer, and Type 2 diabetes.[542]

Insulin resistance and its associated conditions are major contributors to morbidity and mortality worldwide. They significantly increase the risk of premature death, primarily due to cardiovascular complications and Type 2 Diabetes.[543] The healthcare burden of managing these conditions is immense. Emerging evidence suggests that magnesium intake may offer a valuable tool in the fight against insulin resistance, potentially improving outcomes and reducing the burden of related diseases.[473] As the prevalence of insulin resistance continues to rise, a multifaceted approach combining lifestyle interventions and nutritional support will be crucial in mitigating its impact on global health.

In a paper by Kostov K., he states that currently, the most compelling evidence indicates that magnesium deficiency impacts insulin secretion, insulin sensitivity, systemic inflammatory responses, and the activity of key magnesium-dependent enzymes involved in carbohydrate and energy metabolism.[544] We will briefly touch on each one of these.

Insulin Secretion

In magnesium deficiency, decreased intracellular levels of magnesium inhibits the closure and opening of the ATP-sensitive potassium channels.[545] The ATP-sensitive potassium channel is crucial for insulin release from pancreatic beta cells. This disruption affects the coupling between blood glucose levels and the electrical stimulation of beta-cells, leading to an abnormal insulin release. ATP, which is the energy used by our cells, is activated by magnesium. When magnesium binds to ATP the terminal phosphate bond on ATP gets cleaved and this releases energy.[546, 547]

Magnesium ACTIVATES ATP

Magnesium binds to ATP releasing phosphate and liberates its energy

$$ATP + Mg^{2+} \qquad ADP + Phosphate + Mg^{2+} + energy$$

$$Adenosine - P - P - P \rightarrow Adenosine - P - P + P$$

$$\uparrow$$

$$Mg2+ \qquad\qquad + Mg2+$$

$$+ \ Energy$$

Adapted From: Toto and Yucha (1994). 'Magnesium: homeostasis, imbalances, and therapeutic uses.' Critical care nursing clinics of North America, 6(4), 767–783. ATP = adenosine triphosphate, ADP = adenosine diphosphate.

Thus, active ATP should really be thought of as magnesium-ATP. At normal magnesium concentrations, magnesium-ATP levels are sufficient to maintain the proper opening of ATP-sensitive potassium channels. However, in magnesium deficiency, reduced magnesium-ATP levels prevent the opening of these channels, causing prolonged depolarization of the beta-cell membrane and increased insulin release. [544] This was observed in healthy individuals, where those with lower plasma magnesium (0.79

mmol/L) had higher fasting insulin levels (23 µU/mL) compared to those with higher magnesium levels (0.87 or 1.00 mmol/L), who had lower fasting insulin levels (11 µU/mL).[548]

Insulin Sensitivity

Magnesium is crucial for glucose metabolism as it helps with GLUT-4 translocation to the cell membrane to allow glucose into the cell as well as improving the function of the insulin receptor.[549]

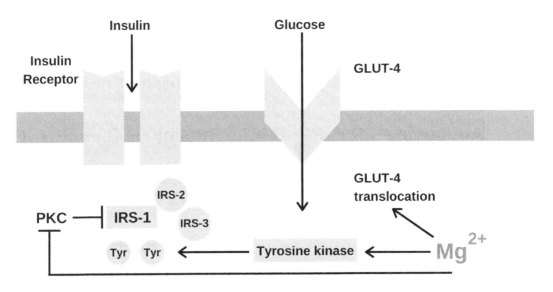

Adapted from Takaya J, Higashino H and Kobayashi Y. Intracellular magnesium and insulin resistance. Magnesium Research. 2004;17(2):126-135.

Low magnesium levels can disrupt the function of many enzymes involved in glucose metabolism and impair insulin receptor activity by increasing the microviscosity of the plasma membrane, thereby reducing insulin sensitivity.[550, 551] The magnesium-ATP complex helps improve insulin sensitivity by regulating the activity of tyrosine kinase in the insulin receptor and promoting the autophosphorylation of the receptor's beta subunit, which then leads to the phosphorylation of its substrates.[544] Insulin receptors are composed of two alpha subunits and two beta subunits with inherent tyrosine kinase activity.[549] Low intracellular magnesium levels can impair the tyrosine kinase activity of these insulin receptors, affecting insulin sensitivity. This intracellular magnesium deficiency may contribute to the development of insulin resistance and hinder glucose entry into cells.[549] Adequate magnesium levels enhance the activity of the insulin receptor tyrosine kinase, which is crucial for the insulin signal transduction.[544]

Magnesium acts as a natural calcium antagonist, helping regulate intracellular calcium levels.[340] Elevated intracellular calcium levels can impair insulin signaling and contribute to insulin resistance. Magnesium modulates the activity of various calcium channels, including voltage-gated calcium channels and receptor-operated calcium channels. By regulating these channels, magnesium helps control the influx of calcium into cells. Excessive calcium influx can activate signaling pathways that negatively impact insulin signaling. Magnesium's regulatory effect on calcium channels helps prevent this dysregulation, thereby supporting insulin sensitivity.[545, 552]

Systemic Inflammatory Responses

Inflammation is a key factor in the development of insulin resistance, involving various cytokines and molecular pathways.[553] Magnesium deficiency exacerbates this by increasing the production of proinflammatory molecules like IL-1β, IL-6, TNF-α, and others, while reducing the activity of antioxidant enzymes such as glutathione peroxidase, superoxide dismutase, and catalase. Increased inflammation and reduced antioxidant levels lead to higher oxidative stress. These changes can contribute to an environment that promotes insulin resistance.[544] The anti-inflammatory and antioxidant effects of magnesium have been well-documented in both preclinical and clinical scientific literature.[2]

Carbohydrate and Energy Metabolism

Magnesium deficiency can limit carbohydrate and energy metabolism because many enzymes in these processes need magnesium or magnesium-ATP to function. In pancreatic beta cells, magnesium directly affects glucokinase activity, which relies on magnesium-ATP.[544] In the liver, magnesium regulates enzymes that are involved in gluconeogenesis. Gluconeogenesis is the process of producing glucose from its own breakdown products (lactate) or from the breakdown products of fats or proteins. These enzymes specifically require magnesium to function properly.[554]

To further support the importance of this mineral, a systematic review was conducted to investigate the effect of magnesium supplementation on insulin resistance in humans. Most of the trials included in the review found that magnesium supplementation improved fasting glucose levels and insulin resistance.[555] A meta-analysis by Simmental-Mendía et al. evaluated the effects of magnesium supplementation on glycemic markers in both diabetic and non-diabetic patients. The study concluded that magnesium supplementation can reduce glucose concentrations and improve insulin resistance, thereby aiding in blood glucose control.[556] Finally in a study done by Cahill, F. et al. they investigated the association between dietary magnesium intake and insulin resistance in normal-weight, overweight and obese individuals along with pre- and post-menopausal women.[557] A total of 2,295 subjects participated in this study. The findings revealed that individuals with the highest dietary magnesium intake had the lowest levels of circulating insulin, HOMA-IR index (used to measure insulin resistance), and HOMA-β (a measure of how well the beta cells in the pancreas produce insulin). In contrast, those with the lowest magnesium intake had the highest levels of these measures, indicating a dose-response effect.[557]

Elevated insulin levels can lead to magnesium depletion, disrupting the body's ability to maintain adequate magnesium stores and impacting overall metabolic health. In a study by Djurhuus, M et al. they infused insulin at different rates in seven healthy volunteers.[558] Compared to baseline, renal magnesium excretion increased by 30% at the lower infusion rate and by 50% at the higher infusion rate. It was concluded that physiological concentrations of insulin enhance renal magnesium excretion, which may partly explain the magnesium depletion observed in hyperinsulinemic states, such as diabetes mellitus, atherosclerosis, hypertension, and obesity.[558]

Skeletal muscle can take up glucose efficiently, especially during physical activity, due to increased insulin sensitivity and the translocation of GLUT4 transporters to the cell membrane.[559] Magnesium helps insulin work better by acting on Akt (regulates glucose and lipid metabolism) and GLUT4, which are proteins involved in insulin signaling and glucose uptake in adipocytes (fat cells).[560] This helps regulate the levels of glucose outside of cells. When magnesium levels are low, it can impair the signaling of Akt and GLUT4 and diminish insulin's ability to stimulate glucose uptake in cells like adipocytes and skeletal muscles.[561]

In summary, magnesium enhances insulin signaling and glucose uptake in adipocytes by acting on both Akt and GLUT4, thereby improving extracellular glucose levels. This increased glucose availability leads to higher glycolysis in adipocytes. Thus, it has been concluded that defects in Akt and GLUT4 signaling due to magnesium deficiency may be the key reason behind the link between low magnesium levels and insulin resistance.[561]

This highlights the importance of maintaining adequate magnesium levels. To summarize, magnesium is crucial for normal insulin secretion and activity, as well as for the optimal functioning of many enzymes involved in glucose and energy metabolism. Magnesium deficiency can lead to beta-cell dysfunction, insulin resistance, reduced glucose tolerance, and, ultimately, the clinical manifestations of type 2 diabetes.

Metabolic Syndrome

Metabolic syndrome is characterized by hyperinsulinemia (high insulin) and underlying insulin resistance, along with several other cardiovascular risk factors.[562] These include impaired glucose regulation, elevated triglyceride levels, reduced high-density lipoprotein (HDL) cholesterol levels, increased blood pressure, and centrally-distributed obesity.[563] The diagnosis of metabolic syndrome is made when an individual exhibits at least three of these five risk factors.[562] Metabolic syndrome is a cluster of conditions that occur together, significantly increasing the risk of heart disease, stroke, and type 2 diabetes.[562]

Metabolic syndrome affects a substantial portion of the global population, with estimates suggesting that nearly one in three adults in the United States has this condition.[564] Its prevalence is rising worldwide, paralleling increases in obesity and sedentary lifestyles. This syndrome has profound impacts on individuals' daily lives, contributing to a range of health issues that diminish quality of life. For example, individuals may experience fatigue, difficulty in managing weight, and increased susceptibility to cardiovascular events, which can lead to frequent medical visits and a reliance on various medications.[564]

The societal impact of metabolic syndrome is significant, as it imposes a considerable burden on healthcare systems due to the associated chronic diseases and their complications. Moreover, it reduces productivity and increases absenteeism in the workplace. Given the strong association between metabolic syndrome and cardiovascular events, cancer, and increased mortality, preventing metabolic syndrome is crucial for public health.[562]

Emerging research suggests that magnesium may be a potential therapeutic option for managing metabolic syndrome. Magnesium plays a crucial role in various bodily functions, including glucose metabolism and insulin signaling.[473] As we have mentioned, adequate magnesium intake has been shown to improve insulin sensitivity, reduce inflammation, and enhance the function of cells involved in glucose uptake. Therefore, magnesium could help mitigate some of the adverse effects associated with metabolic syndrome, potentially offering a simple and cost-effective strategy to improve health outcomes for those affected by this condition.

A growing body of evidence suggests that low serum magnesium levels have been linked to risk factors for metabolic syndrome, including hyperglycemia, hypertension, hypertriglyceridemia, and insulin resistance.[541] Additionally, waist circumference has been found to be independently associated with hypomagnesemia.[565] Furthermore, some studies have indicated that serum magnesium levels are independently associated with metabolic syndrome.[566, 567] A meta-analysis provided compelling evidence that adults with metabolic syndrome have reduced magnesium levels.[568]

Magnesium's protective effects include reducing inflammation, improving glucose and insulin metabolism, enhancing endothelium-dependent vasodilation, and normalizing the lipid profile.[569] We will examine each risk factor for metabolic syndrome and explore the role magnesium plays in mitigating them.

Central Obesity

Obesity has surged globally over the past 50 years, reaching pandemic proportions. According to the World Health Organization, more than 1.9 billion people worldwide are overweight, with over 650 million classified as obese. The prevalence of obesity is notably higher in women, affecting 15% of the population, compared to 11% in men.[570]

Changes in magnesium metabolism have been observed in obese patients, resulting in reduced magnesium levels in serum, plasma, and erythrocytes.[571] A recent meta-analysis found that overweight and obese women with polycystic ovary syndrome had significantly lower magnesium concentrations compared to normal-weight controls.[572] Another population-based study involving 130 healthy adults revealed a significant negative correlation between body weight, waist circumference, and total serum magnesium levels.[573] It should be noted that magnesium deficiency can affect not only obese adults but also children. Research by Hassan et al. showed that overweight and obese children had significantly lower magnesium levels compared to their normal-weight peers, with a strong inverse correlation between serum magnesium levels and body mass index.[574]

Obesity often results from unhealthy diets high in calories but low in essential nutrients, thus leading to magnesium deficiency.[473] Insufficient magnesium intake triggers a pro-inflammatory response in overweight and obese individuals. This intestinal inflammation further hampers micronutrient absorption.[575] A meta-analysis showed that for every 100 mg/day increase in magnesium intake, the overall risk of developing metabolic syndrome was reduced by 17%.[576] They concluded that dietary magnesium intake is inversely associated with the prevalence of metabolic syndrome. A diet high in calcium, fiber or fat can interfere with magnesium absorption in the intestines.[577] Additionally, magnesium deficiency combined with a high-fructose diet induces insulin resistance, hypertension, dyslipidemia, and endothelial activation. It also promotes prothrombotic changes and upregulates markers of inflammation and oxidative stress.[578]

Chronic magnesium deficiency reduces extracellular magnesium levels and increases intracellular calcium concentration, leading to the activation of phagocytic cells and the release of inflammatory cytokines. Animal studies support that subclinical magnesium deficiency can trigger chronic inflammatory reactions in humans by allowing abnormal calcium entry into cells, which promotes the release of inflammatory molecules such as neuropeptides, cytokines, prostaglandins, and leukotrienes. [217] The 30-year longitudinal CARDIA study, involving over 5,000 subjects, found that magnesium intake is inversely associated with obesity and C-reactive protein levels (inflammatory marker).[579] In a study conducted by Guerrero-Romero et al., the link between severe hypomagnesemia and low-grade inflammation in metabolic syndrome was examined. The study included 98 individuals newly diagnosed with metabolic syndrome. Participants were categorized by serum magnesium levels into three groups: severe hypomagnesemia (≤ 1.2 mg/dL), hypomagnesemia ($>1.2-\leq 1.8$ mg/dL), and normal levels (>1.8 mg/dL). Low-grade inflammation was indicated by elevated hsCRP or TNF-alpha levels. Severe hypomagnesemia was found in 21.4% of participants and was strongly associated with increased hsCRP and TNF-alpha levels, while normal magnesium levels were protective.[580] Inflammation is a key underlying mechanism and risk factor for the development of cardiovascular diseases, including coagulation disorders, atherosclerosis, metabolic syndrome, insulin resistance, and diabetes mellitus.[581]

Additionally, appropriate vitamin D levels are crucial as they correlate with magnesium status, especially in obese individuals who often experience vitamin D deficiency. Magnesium is essential for the synthesis and activation of vitamin D, which has protective effects against metabolic disorders.[582] A study by Stokic et al. demonstrated that chronic vitamin D deficiency, combined with low magnesium levels, increases the risk of cardiometabolic disorders in non-diabetic obese individuals, while optimal magnesium levels enhance the protective effects of vitamin D.[583]

Magnesium is needed to ACTIVATE vitamin D

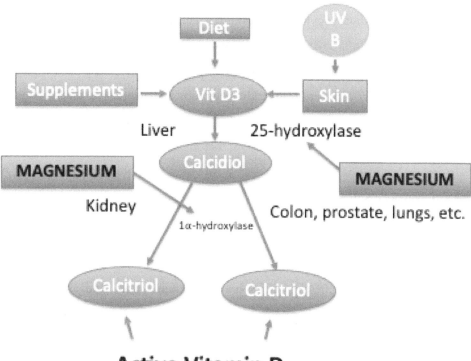

Active Vitamin D

Hypertension

We covered hypertension in detail in Chapter 3 of this book and will revisit it here in the context of its relationship to metabolic syndrome. Hypertension is the most significant independent and modifiable risk factor for coronary diseases such as heart failure, stroke, myocardial infarction, and chronic kidney disease.[584] Alarmingly, about 46% of adults with hypertension are unaware of their condition.[584] Thus, it represents a growing health problem, necessitating new strategies to combat its spread. Observational studies have shown an inverse correlation between magnesium serum levels and dietary intake with hypertension.[585]

A low dietary magnesium intake leading to hypomagnesemia may contribute to the development of hypertension. Magnesium deficiency can cause cell dysfunction and elevate the risk of thrombosis and atherosclerosis. Magnesium helps reduce vascular tone and resistance by releasing nitric oxide from the coronary endothelium and counteracting vasoconstrictor molecules like calcium, bradykinin, angiotensin II, and serotonin.[8] As mentioned before, magnesium acts as a natural calcium channel blocker, inhibiting calcium entry into cells under normal conditions. Calcium influx into smooth muscle cells and cardiomyocytes is essential for their contraction and the regulation of vascular tone. Intracellular levels of calcium and magnesium are regulated by binding to specific proteins and controlled by a calcium-magnesium-ATPase pump and calcium channels. In hypertensive patients, increased calcium and decreased magnesium levels in cell membranes have been observed. This imbalance may increase smooth muscle cell contraction and decrease relaxation, thereby increasing blood pressure.[569] Oxidative stress has also been shown to play a role in raising blood pressure.[586] Additionally, adequate magnesium levels can modulate vascular tone and blood pressure through antioxidant and anti-inflammatory effects, reducing reactive oxygen species formation and limiting vasoconstriction.[569]

Interestingly, insulin can act as both an inflammatory and anti-inflammatory agent. Under normal conditions, insulin stimulates endothelial nitric oxide production, promoting vasorelaxation and reducing inflammation. However, in states of insulin resistance, the insulin-stimulated nitric oxide pathway is selectively impaired. As a result, compensatory hyperinsulinemia can activate the mitogen-activated protein kinase pathway, leading to increased vasoconstriction, inflammation, sodium and water retention, and elevated blood pressure. [587]

Magnesium supplementation as a treatment for hypertension has been shown in numerous clinical studies in humans. A meta-analysis of randomized, double-blind, placebo-controlled trials in both normotensive and hypertensive adults found that magnesium supplementation significantly reduces systolic blood pressure and diastolic blood pressure, along with increasing serum magnesium concentration.[230] Another meta-analysis by Asbaghi et al. showed that while magnesium supplementation did not affect body weight, it significantly reduced systolic blood pressure and diastolic blood pressure in patients with type 2 diabetes mellitus.[588] Additionally, a further meta-analysis involving individuals with insulin resistance, prediabetes, or non-communicable chronic diseases found that magnesium supplementation led to an average reduction of 4.18 mmHg in systolic blood pressure and 2.27 mmHg in diastolic blood pressure.[589]

Elevated Triglycerides and Reduced High-Density Lipoprotein Levels

Increased triglycerides and low levels of high-density lipoprotein (HDL) cholesterol are key components of metabolic syndrome and can elevate the risk of cardiovascular disease and type 2 diabetes.[562] High triglyceride levels are indicative of insulin resistance, which can contribute to the buildup of plaque in the arteries, leading to atherosclerosis and other cardiovascular complications. Low HDL cholesterol, often referred to as "good" cholesterol, further exacerbates this risk, as HDL is responsible for transporting cholesterol away from the arteries and back to the liver for excretion.[590] Together, these lipid abnormalities disrupt normal lipid metabolism and addressing these factors are crucial for reducing the overall risk associated with metabolic syndrome.

Magnesium has been reported to increase HDL cholesterol and reduce LDL cholesterol and triglycerides by inhibiting the action of lecithin cholesterol acyltransferase[591] and HMG-CoA reductase, as well as by enhancing lipoprotein lipase activity.[592] In a 12-week double-blind, placebo-controlled, randomized clinical trial involving 86 participants with prediabetes, it was shown that a daily intake of 250 mg of magnesium significantly increased HDL-cholesterol levels.[593] Additionally, magnesium may decrease the absorption of fatty acids and cholesterol in the intestine by forming an unabsorbable compound, thereby reducing dietary energy intake and potentially aiding in weight management.[594]

Magnesium deficiency can induce hypertriglyceridemia and pro-atherogenic changes in lipoprotein metabolism. This, combined with endothelial dysfunction, enhances platelet aggregation, increasing the risk of thrombotic events.[586]

Impaired Glucose Regulation

Impaired glucose regulation is a key component of metabolic syndrome. When the body is unable to effectively manage blood glucose levels, it can lead to elevated blood sugar and insulin resistance. Over time, this dysregulation can progress to type 2 diabetes, characterized by consistently high blood sugar levels that damage organs and tissues.[473] Additionally, impaired glucose regulation contributes to the development of cardiovascular diseases, as it is often associated with hypertension, abnormal cholesterol levels, and obesity.[562] These interrelated conditions collectively heighten the risk of heart attacks, strokes, and other serious cardiovascular events.

As we have mentioned, higher magnesium levels correspond to greater insulin sensitivity, explaining the improvement in glycemic control indicators after magnesium supplementation. This improvement could be attributed to various mechanisms, including magnesium's influence on insulin receptor activity through enhanced tyrosine kinase phosphorylation.[549] In a study by Guerrero-Romero et al. they found that daily oral magnesium supplementation substantially improved insulin sensitivity by 10% and reduced blood sugar by 37%.[595] Furthermore, a systematic review and meta-analysis of double-blind randomized controlled trials found that magnesium supplementation significantly benefits glucose parameters in individuals with type 2 diabetes and enhances insulin sensitivity in those at high risk of developing diabetes.[596]

Much of what we discussed in the insulin resistance section of this chapter applies here as well. The mechanisms by which magnesium enhances insulin sensitivity and supports glucose uptake are critical to understanding its role in maintaining healthy blood sugar levels.

As evidenced by numerous research studies, magnesium plays a crucial role in mitigating metabolic syndrome by positively influencing its individual components, including glucose metabolism, lipid profiles, weight management and blood pressure regulation. Furthermore, its function as a cofactor for key enzymes involved in insulin signaling underscores its potential as a therapeutic option for preventing and managing metabolic syndrome.

Diabetes

Diabetes mellitus, commonly known as diabetes, is a chronic metabolic disorder characterized by high levels of blood glucose (sugar) due to the body's inability to produce or effectively use insulin. Insulin is a hormone produced by the pancreas that regulates blood sugar levels. There are three main types of diabetes: Type 1, Type 2, and gestational diabetes. Type 1 diabetes is an autoimmune condition where the body's immune system attacks insulin-producing cells in the pancreas, leading to little or no insulin production. Type 2 diabetes, the most prevalent form, occurs when the body becomes resistant to insulin, or the pancreas fails to produce sufficient insulin.[597] Gestational diabetes develops during pregnancy and usually resolves after childbirth, but it can increase the risk of developing Type 2 diabetes later in life.[598]

The symptoms of diabetes can vary depending on the type and severity of the condition. Common symptoms include increased thirst, frequent urination, extreme hunger, unexplained weight loss, fatigue, irritability, blurred vision, slow-healing sores, and frequent infections. In Type 1 diabetes, symptoms can develop quickly over a few weeks or months, while in Type 2 diabetes, they may develop more slowly and be less noticeable initially.[597] Gestational diabetes may not present noticeable symptoms and is often detected through routine prenatal screening.[598]

Diabetes is a growing global health concern, affecting millions of people worldwide. The prevalence of diabetes is increasing in both developed and developing countries, driven by factors such as aging populations, urbanization, unhealthy diets, physical inactivity, and rising obesity rates. Type 2 diabetes accounts for about 90-95% of all diabetes cases, and its prevalence is particularly high in low- and middle-income countries undergoing rapid socio-economic changes.[540]

The causes of diabetes are multifaceted, involving a combination of genetic, environmental, and lifestyle factors. Type 1 diabetes is believed to result from a complex interplay of genetic predisposition and environmental triggers, such as viral infections. Type 2 diabetes is strongly associated with lifestyle factors, including poor diet, lack of physical activity, and obesity. Other risk factors for Type 2 diabetes include age, ethnicity, and certain health conditions such as hypertension and polycystic ovary syndrome (PCOS).[599] Gestational diabetes is primarily influenced by hormonal changes during pregnancy and genetic and lifestyle factors.[598]

The impact of diabetes on society is profound, affecting individuals, families, and healthcare systems. It is a leading cause of morbidity and mortality, contributing to serious health complications such as cardiovascular disease, stroke, kidney failure, nerve damage, and blindness. Diabetes-related complications can significantly reduce quality of life and increase healthcare costs. The economic burden of diabetes is substantial, encompassing direct medical costs for treatment and management, as well as indirect costs related to lost productivity, disability, and premature death.[540, 597] Addressing the diabetes epidemic requires a multifaceted approach. One effective approach involves magnesium which can play a beneficial role in diabetes management. This effective strategy may help mitigate the risk and progression of the disease.

Type 2 diabetes mellitus involves both insulin deficiency and insulin resistance. Hyperglycemia occurs when the body's insulin production cannot keep up with the increased demands due to insulin resistance. Type 2 diabetes is frequently linked to disrupted magnesium balance, with magnesium intake inversely related to type 2 diabetes risk in a dose-dependent manner.[600] Studies have shown a high prevalence of hypomagnesemia in individuals with type 2 diabetes[601], primarily due to low dietary intake, insulin resistance and increased urinary magnesium loss, likely from impaired renal function.[602, 603] Recent findings highlight a strong association between hypomagnesemia and type 2 diabetes progression.[604] Hypomagnesemia in diabetes has also been linked to worse glycemic control, as well as an increased risk of retinopathy, nephropathy, and foot ulcers.[605] While insulin regulates magnesium homeostasis, magnesium also plays a crucial role in post-receptor insulin signaling. This interaction influences glucose metabolism and insulin sensitivity, explaining the inverse relationship between magnesium intake and type 2 diabetes incidence.[606] Magnesium deficiency significantly impacts insulin secretion and may lead to pancreatic beta cell dysfunction in Type 2 diabetes.[544] Magnesium is crucial for glucose-dependent signaling that triggers insulin release. Many glycolytic enzymes and glucokinase (acts as the "glucose sensor" for the pancreas) rely on the magnesium-ATP complex, so low intracellular magnesium levels result in decreased cellular ATP, impairing insulin production.[544]

Reduced intracellular ATP and magnesium-ATP levels disrupt the regulation of ATP-sensitive potassium channels, leading to increased basal insulin secretion and hyperinsulinemia. This chronic insulin exposure contributes to insulin resistance, exacerbated by low-grade inflammation.[544] Additionally, prolonged hyperinsulinemia in insulin resistance increases renal magnesium excretion, perpetuating a vicious cycle of deficiency and resistance.[85] In addition and as mentioned in the insulin resistance section of this chapter, low intracellular magnesium impairs cell responsiveness to insulin by altering the tyrosine-kinase activity of the insulin receptor. This disruption leads to post-receptor insulin resistance and decreases cellular glucose utilization.[544]

Akt, also known as Protein Kinase B, is a protein in cells that helps regulate important processes such as glucose uptake, cell growth, and survival.[607] It plays a key role in regulating the metabolic actions of insulin, such as glucose uptake through GLUT4 mobilization in skeletal muscle and adipose tissue, as well as glycogen and protein synthesis, and lipogenesis.[473] Consequently, lower basal intracellular magnesium levels necessitate higher insulin amounts to metabolize the same glucose load, indicating reduced insulin sensitivity.[608] Based on these findings we can emphasize that insulin action is highly dependent on intracellular magnesium concentration.

Diabetic nephropathy is the leading cause of end-stage renal disease, with about 20% of Type 2 diabetes patients developing this condition over their lifetime.[609] The pathogenesis of diabetic nephropathy involves multiple molecular mechanisms such as activation of polyol and protein kinase C pathways, accumulation of advanced glycation end products, glomerular hyperfiltration, and hypertension.[609] Studies have indicated that low serum magnesium levels can influence the development and progression of diabetic nephropathy.[610] Researchers have concluded that hypomagnesemia is significantly associated with diabetic nephropathy and can serve as a marker for its risk.[610] A study by Prabodh et al., also suggested a link between hypomagnesemia and the onset of diabetic nephropathy.[611] Finally, a study by Guerrero-Romero et al., has shown that low serum magnesium concentrations are linked to a more rapid decline in renal function in Type 2 diabetes patients, predicting the progression to end-stage renal disease in those with diabetic nephropathy.[612]

Chronic high blood glucose levels in diabetes leads to complications due to non-enzymatic glycosylation of proteins and sorbitol accumulation, causing irreversible tissue changes. This results in both microvascular and macrovascular complications, including neuropathy. Diabetic peripheral neuropathy is a prevalent complication of diabetes, affecting about 50% of diabetic patients.[613] It is also a significant independent risk factor for diabetic foot ulcers, which are a leading cause of lower extremity amputation in diabetic patients.[614] Low serum magnesium levels are linked to diabetic foot ulcers.[615] Thus, managing magnesium levels in diabetic patients, whether or not they have foot ulcers, is crucial, and magnesium supplementation can be a beneficial additional treatment. A recent randomized controlled trial showed that 12 weeks of magnesium supplementation in patients with diabetic foot ulcers resulted in improvements in ulcer size and inflammation (serum CRP concentration).[616]

Diabetic macrovascular complications refer to large blood vessel damage caused by diabetes, leading to conditions such as cardiovascular disease, peripheral artery disease, and stroke. These complications, particularly cardiovascular disease, are the leading cause of death among diabetic patients.[597] Studies indicate that even low-normal serum magnesium levels are linked to higher all-cause mortality in individuals with Type 2 diabetes.[617] Research by Agrawal et al. found that low magnesium levels are associated with the oxidation of LDL cholesterol, promoting atherosclerosis and diabetic macrovascular disease.[618] Furthermore, a study done by Wang et al. reported an inverse relationship between serum magnesium and diabetic macrovascular complications, including cardiovascular and peripheral artery diseases.[619]

Insulin resistance is a major factor in the development of Type 2 diabetes mellitus and as discussed earlier it often results from impairments in intracellular insulin signaling.[608] Magnesium has anti-inflammatory effects in adipose tissue, reducing the secretion of inflammatory cytokines such as interleukin-1 (IL-1) and TNF-alpha (TNF-α).[608] Pro-inflammatory cytokines can impair glucose uptake by reducing insulin receptor substrate-1 expression (plays a crucial role in maintaining normal glucose homeostasis), decreasing GLUT4 protein (which facilitates the uptake of glucose into cells) levels as well as reducing Akt activity.[544, 608] Additionally, magnesium serves as a cofactor for ATPases that are crucial in the glycolytic pathway.[8] In a study by Hata, A et al. it was shown that higher magnesium intake was a significant protective factor against the onset of Type 2 diabetes in the general Japanese population.[620] This was particularly true among individuals with insulin resistance, low-grade inflammation, and regular alcohol consumption. Previous research has demonstrated that magnesium supplementation can increase GLUT-4 gene expression and translocation (allowing more glucose into the cell) and suppress gluconeogenesis (endogenous glucose production).[621]

Oxidative stress plays a crucial role in the progression and complications of diabetes. Oxidative stress occurs when reactive oxygen species overwhelm the body's antioxidant defenses, causing damage to cells.[622] Various reactive oxygen species, such as hydrogen peroxide, superoxide radicals, and peroxynitrite, contribute to diabetes by damaging mitochondria, DNA, cells, and proteins.[623] As previously mentioned, oxidative stress and inflammation are linked to magnesium deficiency, which may reduce insulin sensitivity. High levels of free radicals are common in conditions like Type 2 diabetes, hypertension, metabolic syndrome, and aging, all of which are associated with low magnesium levels.[609] Mitochondrial dysfunction and reduced mitochondrial mass are key factors in many aging-related and metabolic diseases like Type 2 diabetes and obesity. DNA damage in the mitochondria leads to more dysfunction, creating a cycle of increased reactive oxygen species production.[609] At the cellular level, magnesium helps by enhancing mitochondrial function, boosting ATP production, lowering reactive oxygen species and intracellular calcium overload, stabilizing mitochondrial membranes, as well as reducing oxidative stress.[624]

Research now shows that changes in gut microbiota contribute to systemic low-grade inflammation.[625] Studies suggest that both the structure and diversity of gut microbiota are reduced and altered in people with impaired glucose regulation and Type 2 diabetes.[626] Modifying gut microbiota through diet is an emerging strategy for preventing and treating Type 2 diabetes. Magnesium supplementation can help reshape the microbiota, as it has been shown to impact microbial composition and function in obese subjects.[627] This research shows that ensuring sufficient dietary intake of magnesium may benefit intestinal microbiota composition and host metabolism, potentially aiding in the prevention of metabolic issues linked to metabolic syndrome and Type 2 diabetes. However, more research is needed to fully understand the role of magnesium in this area.

During pregnancy, hormones such as estrogen, progesterone, human chorionic somatomammotropin, prolactin, and cortisol increase insulin resistance. If there isn't enough insulin sensitivity or enough insulin produced to maintain normal blood sugar levels, gestational diabetes develops.[628] Gestational diabetes increases both maternal and fetal morbidity. Gestational diabetic women often face magnesium deficiency due to increased magnesium loss out the urine and reduced intestinal absorption caused by iron supplements. Hyperglycemia in these women leads to an enlarged placenta, driven by the fetal pancreas's increased insulin secretion, a potent growth hormone in utero. This enlarged placenta then produces excess steroid hormones, further reducing magnesium absorption.[628] In a very recent meta-analysis of randomized controlled trials it was found that magnesium supplementation for gestational diabetes significantly reduced fasting plasma glucose by 7.33 mg/dL (95% CI: -7.64 to -7.02 mg/dL, P < 0.00001) and improved insulin resistance (HOMA-IR) by 0.99 (95% CI: -1.76 to -0.22, P = 0.01) compared to the control intervention. It was concluded that magnesium supplementation may be effective for the treatment of gestational diabetes without taking insulin treatment.[629] To further support this, data from four randomized controlled trials looking at the effect of magnesium supplementation on pregnancy outcomes in gestational diabetes patients showed significant improvements in glucose metabolism, insulin sensitivity, as well as total antioxidant capacity.[630]

Supplementation with magnesium has shown promise in benefiting diabetes mellitus and its associated complications, as evidenced by both human and animal studies. Oral magnesium supplementation has demonstrated improvements in insulin secretion and sensitivity, lipid profile, metabolic control, and inflammatory status among patients with Type 2 diabetes mellitus and hypomagnesemia.[609] A meta-analysis of randomized, double-blind, controlled trials showed that oral magnesium supplementation (360 mg per day) for 4-16 weeks can effectively lower fasting plasma glucose levels and increase HDL cholesterol in Type 2 diabetes patients.[631] Other studies have shown that magnesium supplementation improves fasting and postprandial glucose levels as well as reduces C-reactive protein levels in prediabetic patients with hypomagnesemia.[541] Seven cohort studies (encompassing 24,388 persons/year) unequivocally demonstrated that magnesium intake is linked to a reduced risk of developing Type 2 diabetes.[632] In a trial involving 47 hypomagnesemic Type 2 diabetes patients, daily administration of 336 mg of magnesium resulted in notable reductions in tumor necrosis factor-α (an inflammatory cytokine) and 8-isoprostane concentrations (marker of oxidative stress).[633] Meta-analyses have indicated significant associations between magnesium status and Type 2 diabetes risk in Asian populations, with a 100 mg/day increase in dietary magnesium linked to an 8–13% decrease in Type 2 diabetes risk.[634] We must keep in mind that most of the body's magnesium is intracellular, suggesting that cellular concentrations should be assessed alongside serum levels in patients with Type 2 diabetes.[633] Further research is needed to ascertain the efficacy of magnesium supplementation in managing diabetes and its complications, given that serum magnesium concentration may not accurately reflect intracellular magnesium status.

In summary, oral magnesium supplements seem beneficial for individuals with Type 2 diabetes, helping to correct magnesium deficiencies, improve insulin resistance, reduce oxidative stress, and alleviate systemic inflammation.

Conclusion

Obesity, Type 2 diabetes, and metabolic syndrome are interconnected conditions marked by chronic low-grade inflammation and insulin resistance linked in part to magnesium deficiency. In these metabolic disorders, inadequate magnesium levels from poor diets foster a pro-inflammatory environment that worsens metabolic dysfunction. Magnesium supplementation appears to interrupt this harmful cycle.

As we have mentioned, magnesium plays a crucial role in metabolic health, offering significant benefits for conditions like insulin resistance, metabolic syndrome, and Type 2 diabetes. Its role in glucose metabolism, insulin sensitivity, and inflammatory regulation makes it a simple yet effective treatment option. Magnesium deficiency is prevalent among individuals with these conditions, exacerbating their symptoms and complications. Supplementing with magnesium can address this deficiency, helping to improve fasting and postprandial glucose levels, enhance insulin sensitivity, and reduce markers of inflammation. As we have shown, clinical studies have demonstrated that oral magnesium supplements can lead to measurable improvements in glycemic control, inflammation, and lipid profiles, underscoring its potential as a therapeutic adjunct.

Incorporating magnesium supplementation into treatment plans for insulin resistance, metabolic syndrome, and Type 2 diabetes should be strongly considered by healthcare providers. Its ease of use, affordability, and safety profile make it an accessible intervention for many patients. Additionally, the potential for magnesium to improve overall metabolic function and mitigate the risk of complications like neuropathy and cardiovascular disease highlights its importance in comprehensive metabolic health management. As research continues to uncover the mechanisms and benefits of magnesium, its role in preventing and managing metabolic disorders will likely become even more pronounced, solidifying its place as a key component in the fight against these prevalent and debilitating conditions.

Chapter 6: Magnesium for Bone and Kidney Health

Optimal bone health is essential for overall well-being. This includes the strength, density, and structural integrity of bones. It entails maintaining bones that are resilient and capable of withstanding daily stresses without breaking or fractures. Proper bone health affects individuals of all ages and is fundamental to mobility, posture, and protection of vital organs.[635]

Bone health significantly influences an individual's quality of life. Healthy bones allow for smooth and efficient movement, participation in physical activities, and performance of daily tasks without discomfort. Conversely, poor bone health can lead to a range of complications, including pain, deformities, and a heightened risk of fractures. These issues can severely impact an individual's independence and overall lifestyle.[635]

Bone health is critical across the lifespan. Children and adolescents require strong bones for growth and development, while adults need to maintain bone density to prevent deterioration. Older adults are particularly susceptible to bone health issues due to the natural decline in bone mass with age. Women, especially post-menopausal women, are at a higher risk due to hormonal changes that accelerate bone loss.[636]

Poor bone health can lead to conditions such as osteopenia and osteoporosis, which are characterized by fragile bones and an increased risk of fractures. Osteoporotic fractures, particularly hip fractures, are associated with significant morbidity, including chronic pain and disability. These fractures can also lead to increased mortality, particularly in older adults, due to complications such as infections and reduced mobility post-fracture.[636]

Other conditions that can impair bone health include Paget's disease (a chronic disorder that can result in enlarged and misshapen bones), osteomalacia (softening of the bones due to a deficiency of vitamin D or calcium), and rickets (a similar condition to osteomalacia but occurring in children, leading to bone deformities).[637]

Maintaining good bone health is vital for a high quality of life. It ensures that individuals can stay active, avoid injuries, and live independently for as long as possible. Adequate nutrition, regular exercise, and lifestyle modifications such as avoiding smoking and excessive alcohol consumption all play a crucial role in preserving bone health.

Emerging research suggests that magnesium may serve as an adjunctive treatment for bone health and related conditions. Magnesium plays a key role in bone formation and influences the activities of osteoblasts and osteoclasts, the cells responsible for bone formation and resorption, respectively.[638] Ensuring adequate magnesium intake can help support bone density and overall skeletal health.

Magnesium and Bone Health

About 60% of the body's magnesium is stored in the bones. One-third of this skeletal magnesium is found in the cortical bone, either on the surface of hydroxyapatite or in the hydration shell around the crystal.[12, 638] Hydroxyapatite is a mineral that makes up a significant part of bone, giving it strength and structure.[639] The hydration shell refers to a layer of water molecules that surrounds the crystal.[640] Magnesium is found in this watery layer around the hydroxyapatite. This magnesium acts as a reservoir, helping to maintain normal extracellular magnesium levels.[12] Bone surface magnesium levels are connected to serum magnesium levels, meaning that as magnesium intake increases, so does the magnesium on the bone surface.[638] Experimental magnesium deficiency leads to a 30-40% decrease in bone magnesium content.[12]

Most of the bone magnesium is embedded within the apatite crystals which is released only during bone resorption. Besides its structural role in bones, magnesium is crucial for all living cells, including bone-forming osteoblasts and bone-resorbing osteoclasts.[638] Inside cells, magnesium is vital for various functions. As we have mentioned it is essential for making and activating ATP, the primary energy source for cells, and acts as a cofactor for hundreds of enzymes involved in the synthesis of lipids, proteins, and nucleic acids.[641] Magnesium also stabilizes cell membranes, counteracts calcium, and functions as a signal transducer. Therefore, any disruption in magnesium balance can significantly affect cell and tissue functions.[638]

Osteoporosis

Osteoporosis is a complex condition marked by a significant reduction in bone mass and deterioration of bone microarchitecture. Normally, bones undergo constant remodeling through the coordinated actions of osteoclasts, which break down bone tissue, and osteoblasts, which build and mineralize new bone.[642] Osteoporosis arises when there is an imbalance in this process, favoring bone resorption over bone formation. This leads to a decrease in bone mass, increasing the risk of fractures, especially in the hip and spine. Such fractures can cause severe pain, disability, and even death.[642]

Diagnosis of osteoporosis typically involves a bone density test, such as a dual-energy X-ray absorptiometry (DEXA) scan, which measures the amount of bone mineral in specific areas of the skeleton.[643] A T-score is calculated to describe the density of bones, usually at the spine and hip, and compares bone strength to an average young adult. A T-score below -2.5 standard deviations indicates osteoporosis, while a score between -1 and -2.5 standard deviations indicates osteopenia or low bone density. Normal bone density is within 1 standard deviation of a young adult average.[643]

Osteoporosis impacts millions globally, with postmenopausal women being the most affected group.[638] Estrogen plays a crucial role in maintaining bone strength by slowing down the natural process of bone breakdown. When estrogen levels drop during menopause, this protective effect diminishes, leading to a rapid increase in bone loss.[644] In the United States alone, over 40 million people are at risk of osteoporosis due to low bone mass.[645] By 2050, Europe is projected to have more than 30 million people dealing with osteoporosis. This condition is closely linked to aging, making it a significant health issue as the aging population is expected to double in the next decade, posing a substantial financial burden on healthcare systems.[638]

A strong association has been identified between bone density and magnesium intake.[638] It is essential to consider this mineral when examining osteoporosis as its imbalance can impact the structure and strength of bones.[646] Multiple studies across various species have shown that a diet low in magnesium contributes to osteoporosis. Animals with magnesium deficiency have brittle, fragile bones, with detectable microfractures in the trabeculae and significantly compromised mechanical properties.[638] Trabecular bone, also known as cancellous bone, is a porous type of bone made up of a network of trabeculated bone tissue.[647] As a result, it is evident that a magnesium-deficient diet negatively impacts peri-implant cortical bone, significantly reducing tibial cortical thickness.[638] Tibial cortical thickness is a reliable method for evaluating osteoporosis when dual-energy X-ray absorptiometry is unavailable.[648]

In another study the authors studied sixty patients with osteoporosis to assess serum and red blood cell magnesium and calcium levels. Among them, thirty-three had senile osteoporosis, eighteen had postmenopausal osteoporosis, and nine had corticosteroid-induced osteoporosis. The first two groups exhibited signs of chronic magnesium deficiency, while the third group showed a trend of low serum calcium levels. These findings underscore the crucial role of magnesium in bone metabolism disorders.[649]

In a study by Castiglioni, S. et al. it was revealed that there are multiple direct and indirect mechanisms that contribute to the impact of low magnesium on bone density.[638] It is also important to note that the mechanisms underlying the effects of magnesium deficiency on bone health in humans are similar to those observed in experimental models. Magnesium deficiency results in hypomagnesemia, which is partially countered by the release of surface magnesium from bones. Under the direct mechanism, it has been demonstrated that in magnesium-deficient animals, newly formed apatite crystals are larger and more structured, leading to changes in bone stiffness. Additionally, low magnesium intake slows down cartilage and bone differentiation as well as matrix calcification. In rodents who had magnesium deficiency it was shown that reduced bone formation was partly due to decreased osteoblastic (formation of bone) activity. Histomorphometry also revealed a reduction in the number of osteoblasts as well as lower levels of osteoblastic function markers, such as alkaline phosphatase and osteocalcin. Conversely, the number of osteoclasts (bone cells that break down bone tissue) increased.[638, 650] Another study found that a deficiency in magnesium is inversely proportional to the number of osteoclasts generated from bone marrow precursors. The lower the extracellular magnesium concentration, the higher the number of osteoclasts.[651]

In addition to directly affecting bone structure and cells, magnesium deficiency indirectly impacts bone health by disrupting the balance of two key regulators of calcium, parathyroid hormone and 1,25(OH)2-vitamin D, leading to low calcium levels.[638] Magnesium also heightens the sensitivity of parathyroid cells to calcium.[652] Parathyroid hormone activates vitamin D helping to improve calcium absorption. Low magnesium levels impair parathyroid hormone secretion and reduces organ responsiveness to parathyroid hormone in part due to decreased cyclic AMP production by adenylate cyclase, which requires magnesium as a cofactor.[638, 641] Reduced parathyroid hormone secretion or an impaired response to it lowers 1,25(OH)2-vitamin D levels in the blood.[638] Magnesium deficiency reduces the activity of the enzyme 25-hydroxycholecalciferol-1-hydroxylase, which is essential for vitamin D activation.[638] Magnesium aids in the activation of vitamin D, which regulates calcium and phosphate balance, influencing bone growth and maintenance. In fact, all enzymes that metabolize vitamin D require magnesium as a cofactor for their reactions in the liver and kidneys.[646]

Another indirect impact on bone health is inflammation and oxidative stress. Low magnesium levels promote inflammation.[217] It has been shown that inflammation and bone loss are connected through various molecular pathways.[653] In magnesium-deficient rodents, the levels of inflammatory cytokines, such as TNFα, IL-1, and IL-6, rise in both the blood and the bone marrow. These cytokines increase the activity of osteoclasts (cells that break down bone) while inhibiting osteoblasts (cells that build bone), further perpetuating inflammation. Additionally, magnesium deficiency causes high levels of substance P, which not only boosts the secretion of pro-inflammatory cytokines but also stimulates osteoclast activity in bone.[638, 654] Substance P is a neuropeptide that acts as a neurotransmitter and modulator, playing a role in pain perception and inflammation.[654] Magnesium restriction also leads to oxidative stress due to increased inflammation and reduced antioxidant defenses. This oxidative stress enhances osteoclast activity and suppresses osteoblast function, contributing to further bone loss.[638]

In postmenopausal women, low magnesium intake is associated with faster bone loss and lower bone mineral density. The Framingham Heart Study found a 2% increase in trochanteric bone mineral density for every 100 mg of magnesium consumed by women.[655] The prospective cohort study of 73,684 postmenopausal women from the Women's Health Initiative Observational Study examined the relationship between magnesium intake, bone mineral density, and fracture incidence. The study found that lower daily magnesium intake was associated with lower baseline bone mineral density of the total hip and whole body. Specifically, women who consumed more than 422.5 mg of magnesium per day had a 3% higher hip bone mineral density and a 2% higher whole-body bone mineral density compared to those consuming less than 206.5 mg per day.[655] In a study by Chang, J. et al. it was found that postmenopausal women with osteoporosis have lower serum magnesium levels.[656]

Magnesium directly influences the mineralization process by inhibiting the growth of hydroxyapatite crystals in solution. Larger mineral crystals can make bones brittle and less able to bear normal loads.[12] Magnesium binds to the surface of apatite crystals, slowing down their formation and growth. Postmenopausal women with osteoporosis and magnesium deficiency have been found to have larger an crystals in their trabecular bone.[638]

Studies in postmenopausal women have highlighted estrogen's crucial role in the development of osteoporosis. Estrogen deficiency accelerates bone resorption rather than decreasing new bone formation, leading to significant bone loss.[657] Estrogen supplementation in older women can slow this decline by reducing the rate of bone remodeling and minimizing bone loss during each cycle. Estrogen also enhances magnesium utilization and uptake by soft tissues and bones, which may partly explain the resistance to heart disease and osteoporosis in younger women.[657] Therefore, the role of estrogen in preventing osteoporosis in aging women may be partly due to its effect on magnesium metabolism.

As we have mentioned, magnesium plays a crucial role in vitamin D activation. Magnesium is essential for maintaining bone health, particularly in postmenopausal women and individuals with osteoporosis.[657] Previous studies have demonstrated that the activities of three major enzymes regulating 25(OH)D concentrations, 25-hydroxylase, 1α-hydroxylase, and 24-hydroxylase as well as vitamin D binding protein, are dependent on magnesium. Magnesium deficiency results in reduced levels of 1,25-dihydroxyvitamin D [1,25(OH)2D] and an impaired parathyroid hormone response. This deficiency has been implicated in magnesium-dependent, vitamin D–resistant rickets.[658] Magnesium deficiency is more prevalent in those with low vitamin D levels, affecting calcium absorption and bone health. Magnesium deficiency significantly impacts vitamin D metabolism, highlighting the importance of sufficient magnesium intake for maintaining bone health, especially in postmenopausal women and individuals at high risk for osteoporosis.[657]

The Interaction Between Calcium and Magnesium

Dietary factors significantly influence age-related loss of bone density and skeletal muscle mass. Calcium is essential for bone health, but magnesium also plays a crucial role in mitigating bone density loss.[657] Dietary magnesium can help slow the age-related decline in skeletal muscle mass, which is a risk factor for osteoporosis, falls, fractures, frailty, and mortality. A decrease in magnesium-rich soils and magnesium-poor vegetables, nuts, and legumes has led to inadequate magnesium consumption and chronic deficiencies.[657] Calcium metabolism is vital for bone turnover, and deficiencies in calcium and vitamin D impair bone deposition. Clinical trials have shown that supplementing calcium and vitamin D in older individuals can decrease bone resorption, increase bone density, reduce fractures, and lower the risk of falling.[659]

Parathyroid hormone secretion happens in response to low calcium levels. This leads to increased bone resorption to maintain adequate blood calcium. Conversely, calcitonin, a hormone produced by the thyroid, promotes bone deposition, and reduces serum calcium levels. Magnesium can also reduce parathyroid hormone secretion in low calcium conditions. Restoring magnesium levels in magnesium-depleted individuals can naturally correct low calcium and parathyroid hormone levels without additional calcium supplementation.[657]

Osteoporosis is particularly concerning among the elderly because insufficient magnesium intake leads to excessive calcium release from bones, exacerbating bone fragility and increasing the risk of fractures and falls. Dietary magnesium intake is low in the United States, especially among the elderly and ethnic minorities.[660] High calcium intake can hinder magnesium retention, and low magnesium levels can cause excess calcium excretion. The optimal calcium-to-magnesium ratio is 2–2.8, but since the 1970s, increased calcium consumption in the United States has raised this ratio above 3.0. A balanced intake of these nutrients is crucial for bone health and preventing osteoporosis.[657] Ditmar and Steidl noted that magnesium is crucial for bone matrix formation and mineralization.[661] The rise in magnesium deficiency, due to decreasing levels in soil, food, and water, is a major cause of the increasing rates of osteoporosis in developed countries. Therefore, magnesium should be a central component in both the treatment and prevention of osteoporosis.

Magnesium And Skeletal Metabolism

Magnesium is an essential component of bone, making up 0.5-1% of bone ash. It plays a significant role in bone and mineral metabolism through its effects on hormones and direct impact on bone itself. It has been shown that magnesium depletion negatively impacts all phases of bone metabolism. It has also been shown that decreased bone magnesium has been found in patients with alcoholism, diabetes, and osteoporosis.[662] Furthermore, in a study by Fatemi, S. et al., it was found that mild magnesium depletion can impair mineral homeostasis and may be a risk factor for osteoporosis in conditions such as chronic alcoholism and diabetes mellitus, where both magnesium deficiency and osteoporosis are common.[663]

In a study conducted by Rude, RK et al., they looked at the effect of magnesium intake of 25% of the nutrient requirement on bone and mineral metabolism in a rat model.[664] They specifically assessed its impact on bone mass, calcium metabolism, and inflammatory cytokine presence in bone. The study revealed a significant increase (138-150%) in the immunocytochemical localization of TNF-alpha (inflammatory cytokine) in osteoclasts. This rise in TNF-alpha levels may be linked to elevated substance P levels, which were found to increase from 179% to 432%. These findings indicate that a magnesium intake of 25% of the nutrient requirement in rats may lead to reduced bone mass, possibly through heightened release of substance P and TNF-alpha.[664] In other words, if we transfer this data (25% nutrient requirement of magnesium) a magnesium intake of around 75 mg per day and 100 mg per day in women and men, respectively, may lead to lower bone mass. Another study looked at 50% nutrient requirement of dietary magnesium on bone and mineral metabolism in the rat. Their data also showed a decreased bone mineral content and reduced volume in the distal femur.[665] This reduction of dietary magnesium intake is a level comparable to that seen in a significant portion of the population, suggesting that low magnesium intake may contribute to osteoporosis. What this suggests is that a magnesium intake of around 150 mg per day in women and 200 mg per day in men may lead to reduced bone mineral density and bone volume. Deficiencies in other nutrients like calcium could exacerbate this effect. [78]

To test the hypothesis that magnesium deficiency alters initial mineralization and bone properties, a study by Boskey, AL. et al. compared the bones of rats on a magnesium deficient diet to those of rats on a magnesium supplemented diet.[666] The results showed that short-term magnesium deficiency in growing rats led to a significant decrease in trabecular bone volume and mineral content in the metaphysis. The magnesium deficient rats also had reduced osteocalcin levels (a marker of bone formation) and their bone lipid was more easily extracted. Mechanically, the femurs of magnesium deficient rats showed a significant decrease in maximum three-point bend strength. These findings support the hypothesis that short-term magnesium deficiency impacts the pattern of bone mineral formation.[666]

Magnesium is crucial for normal bone formation and remodeling, but not much is known about the biomechanical function of the bone. A study compared the femurs of male rats fed either adequate or deficient magnesium diets.[667] Magnesium deficient rats exhibited slow growth, poor food utilization, and significantly reduced magnesium levels in serum and femur ash. Their femurs were shorter but similar in weight and diameter to those of the control group. These shorter bones had less dry matter and ash (with higher calcium content per gram), more moisture, and significantly reduced bone strength. Although the modulus of elasticity was unaffected, magnesium deficient bones supported lighter loads at the yield point and at fracture, with decreased stresses even after adjusting for body size. These findings highlight the importance of magnesium in maintaining the biomechanical properties of bone.[667]

Physical activity plays a crucial role in bone mineralization. It has been shown that individuals with low magnesium intake experience accelerated bone mass loss.[668] A study conducted in Portugal examined 17 elite swimmers of both genders to assess the association between magnesium intake, bone mineral density and lean soft tissue. Energy and nutrient intake were assessed over a seven-day period and it was found that magnesium, phosphorus, and vitamin D were significantly below the recommended daily allowance. The study confirmed that magnesium intake was a significant predictor of both bone density and lean tissue, emphasizing the importance of adequate magnesium intake among young athletes participating in low-impact sports to support optimal bone mineralization during growth.[668]

Insulin-dependent diabetes mellitus is a chronic metabolic disorder that can lead to changes in bone metabolism (osteopenia) and disrupt mineral homeostasis, particularly during growth.[669] Factors contributing to diabetic osteopenia include metabolic acidosis, hypocalcemia, insulin deficiency, and possibly hypomagnesemia and hypoparathyroidism.[670] The reduction in bone mineral content among type 1 diabetics is most significant in patients who developed the disease during childhood or adolescence, have ceased beta-cell function, require high insulin doses, and experience poor glucose regulation.[670] It has been shown that the disrupted parathyroid hormone-vitamin D axis in this condition can be reversed by normalizing magnesium serum levels through oral supplementation.[669] In a study examining 23 children with insulin-dependent diabetes mellitus (average age 9.4 years) it was found that they had lower levels of serum calcium (both total and ionized), magnesium, intact parathyroid hormone, calcitriol, and osteocalcin compared to healthy controls.[671] The children were given oral magnesium (6 mg/kg daily) for up to 60 days, which significantly increased the levels of these minerals and hormones to normal values. A low-calcium diet test showed that during magnesium deficiency, the children had a significantly lower response in parathyroid hormone and calcitriol levels. After magnesium supplementation, these responses were similar to those of the control group. This study suggests that magnesium deficiency plays a crucial role in disrupting mineral balance in children with insulin-dependent diabetes mellitus.[671]

Magnesium Supplementation and Bone Health

Studies on magnesium supplementation for bone health primarily focus on postmenopausal women. In a randomized controlled trial with 20 postmenopausal osteoporotic women, 10 women received a daily oral dose of 1,830 mg of magnesium citrate for 30 days.[672] The supplemented group showed significant improvements, e.g., reduced serum parathyroid hormone levels, increased serum osteocalcin levels (marker of bone formation), and decreased urinary deoxypyridinoline levels (marker of bone break down). Deoxypyridinoline, a cross linked product of collagen molecules found in bone, is excreted in urine during bone degradation and is considered a marker of bone turnover.[673]

Another study in Israel followed 54 women for 2 years. Initially, 31 women received 250 mg of magnesium, gradually increasing to 750 mg per day for 6 months, then maintaining at 250 mg for 18 months.[674] The treated group saw significant increases in bone density after one and two years, while untreated women experienced a decrease. Magnesium therapy prevented fractures and increased bone density in 71% of participants.[674]

The importance of magnesium supplementation in menopausal women is well-established, but its benefits for younger individuals, even those without magnesium deficiency, are also worth exploring. In Austria, a study involving 24 men aged 27–36 examined how moderate oral magnesium supplementation affects bone turnover rates over 30 days. The participants were divided into two groups: 12 men took a daily oral dose of magnesium (15 mmol) in a powder form, providing 169 mg of magnesium carbonate and 196 mg of magnesium oxide, dissolved in water, and consumed in the early afternoon with a 2-hour fasting period before and after. The other 12 men, serving as controls, drank a glass of water daily in the afternoon after a 2-hour fast. The results showed that magnesium supplementation significantly reduced serum parathyroid hormone levels and lowered biochemical markers of bone formation and resorption within 1–5 days, indicating that magnesium suppresses bone turnover.[675] A review paper concluded that all interventional studies testing magnesium in humans (at a dose of 250-1,800 mg per day) showed benefits for improving bone mineral density and reducing fracture risk.[676]

Given the role of magnesium in proper bone growth, studies have been conducted on teenagers, particularly females. Carpenter, TO. et al. performed a one-year, double-blind, randomized, placebo-controlled study on 50 teenage girls. They were divided into two groups: 23 girls took magnesium oxide supplements (300 mg of elemental magnesium per day), while 27 girls took a placebo (methylcellulose powder). The magnesium group showed a significant increase in hip bone mineral content and a slight (though not significant) increase in lumbar spinal bone mineral content.[677] Another study in Salt

Lake City, Utah, explored the combined effects of magnesium and other minerals on bone development in pre-adolescent girls. In this study, 81 girls with an average age of 12 were divided into two groups for one year. One group of 38 girls took a chewable vitamin/mineral supplement (800 mg of calcium, 400 mg of magnesium, and 400 IU of vitamin D3 daily), while the other group of 43 girls took a placebo. The supplement group experienced a net gain in trabecular bone mineral density of 1.41%, compared to a statistically significant decline of -0.94% in the placebo group. Additionally, after 12 months, the increase in trabecular bone mineral content was greater in the supplemented group (5.83%) compared to the placebo group (0.69%).[678]

Conclusion on Magnesium and Bone Health

The value and benefits of magnesium in maintaining and enhancing bone health are substantial. Optimizing magnesium intake may be an effective and low-cost preventive measure against osteoporosis, particularly in individuals with documented magnesium deficiency. As discussed, magnesium is essential for various physiological processes that contribute to bone formation and maintenance, including the regulation of calcium levels and the support of bone mineral density. Given its multifaceted role, magnesium supplementation emerges as a vital strategy for supporting bone health, preventing bone-related disorders, and promoting overall skeletal strength and resilience.

Magnesium and Kidney Health - Introduction

Kidney health is vital to overall well-being. The kidneys play a crucial role in filtering waste products, balancing electrolytes, and regulating blood pressure. Diseases affecting the kidneys, such as chronic kidney disease, kidney stones, and infections like pyelonephritis, are increasingly prevalent worldwide.[679] Chronic kidney disease affects millions globally, with significant morbidity and mortality implications due to its progressive nature and associated complications such as cardiovascular disease and kidney failure.[680]

Maintaining optimal kidney function is essential for preventing systemic complications and maintaining overall health. Healthy kidneys contribute to the regulation of blood pressure, production of red blood cells, and activation of vitamin D, crucial for bone health. Impaired kidney function not only leads to accumulation of toxins in the body but also increases the risk of cardiovascular events and premature death.[679]

The research suggests that magnesium may offer therapeutic benefits in supporting kidney health. Magnesium's role in reducing inflammation, preventing kidney stone formation, and potentially slowing the progression of chronic kidney disease through its effects on blood pressure regulation and glucose metabolism is promising. We are going to explore magnesium's mechanisms regarding kidney health and its potential as a preventive or therapeutic option in kidney-related disorders.

Magnesium and Kidney Function

Kidney function is crucial for long-term health, and its decline with age significantly impacts quality of life. As kidneys age, their ability to function well decreases, increasing the risk of acute kidney injury and chronic kidney disease.[681]

In healthy adults, maintaining magnesium balance primarily involves regulating renal magnesium excretion to match intestinal absorption. This balance is essential to keep the body's magnesium levels within physiological ranges. Consequently, any factors that disrupt this process can impair magnesium metabolism, with hypomagnesemia being the most frequent result. Some of the factors that can disrupt magnesium balance include caffeine intake, alcohol consumption, medications (thiazides, proton pump inhibitors etc.), plasma calcium and magnesium, diet content (sodium, potassium, calcium), hormones (parathyroid hormone and calcitonin) and blood volume.[681]

The primary factors influencing magnesium reabsorption by the kidneys are fluctuations in calcium and magnesium levels and blood volume. These variations affect the kidney's reabsorption of water and solutes, including magnesium. Specifically, hypervolemia, also known as fluid overload, reduces magnesium reabsorption, while hypovolemia (low fluid in the body) enhances it.[682] Additionally, both hypermagnesemia and hypercalcemia inhibit magnesium reabsorption in the loop of Henle by activating the calcium-sensing receptor.

Parathyroid hormone and other hormones that activate the cAMP pathway promote calcium reabsorption in the kidney. While no hormones specifically regulate magnesium, both parathyroid hormone and calcitonin are known to positively influence magnesium balance.[681]

Magnesium and Chronic Kidney Disease

Chronic kidney disease is a significant public health concern, impacting around 13% of adults in the U.S. It is a major risk factor for progressing to end-stage renal disease, cardiovascular disease, and it increases mortality.[683] Magnesium's clinical importance in medicine has grown in recent years, particularly among individuals with chronic kidney disease, given its impact on vascular calcification and mineral metabolism.[684] Chronic kidney disease is a long-term condition characterized by the gradual loss of kidney function over time. It develops when the kidneys become damaged and can no longer efficiently filter waste products and excess fluids from the blood.[685] This damage can result from various factors, including high blood pressure, diabetes, and other chronic conditions that place strain on the kidneys. As chronic kidney disease progresses, waste products and fluids build up in the body, leading to complications such as cardiovascular disease, anemia, and bone disorders.[680] Early stages of chronic kidney disease may present with few or no symptoms, making regular screening and early detection crucial for managing the disease and slowing its progression.[680, 685]

In chronic kidney disease there can be a tendency toward hypermagnesemia. This can vary with the disease's severity. In chronic kidney disease stages 1 through 3, the kidneys can compensate for reduced function by increasing fractional magnesium excretion, keeping magnesium levels normal. However, in advanced chronic kidney disease (stages 4–5), these compensatory mechanisms may become inadequate, such that overt hypermagnesemia can occur in those with a creatinine clearance < 10 ml/min.[686] Patients with end-stage renal disease undergoing dialysis typically maintain normal magnesium levels but they also can experience hypomagnesemia. This can be attributed to dietary factors, medication side effects or the magnesium concentration in the dialysate (fluid that is used in dialysis to adjust the extracellular fluid composition and to maintain body homeostasis). In addition, chronic kidney disease patients often have reduced intestinal magnesium absorption compared to healthy individuals. The impaired magnesium absorption appears to be linked to the non-functioning kidney's inability to produce the active metabolite of vitamin D.[687]

Studies show that chronic kidney disease patients with low magnesium levels are more likely to develop vascular calcification, increasing their risk of cardiovascular issues and mortality during dialysis treatment. Additionally, hypomagnesemia is often seen in kidney transplant patients due to the immunosuppressive drugs used to prevent graft failure. Some research also links low magnesium levels after transplantation to the development of new-onset diabetes.[681]

As we have mentioned before, there is a decline in magnesium blood levels with aging. However, it is unclear if this is due to the natural aging process or related to diseases, medications and kidney function problems that come with age.[688] Numerous studies have shown that globally, dietary intake of magnesium is frequently inadequate or insufficient.[1]

For individuals without kidney disease, eating a diet rich in essential nutrients may help prevent kidney failure.[689] There are distinct health consequences associated with low magnesium levels, and this holds true for kidney health as well, where reduced magnesium can impact renal function. In a study by Maier, J. A. et al. they concluded that low magnesium levels directly contribute to endothelial dysfunction by creating an environment that promotes inflammation, blood clot formation, and plaque buildup in arteries.[690] This may play a significant role in the development of cardiovascular disease. Alterations in heart function can cause kidney damage by reducing the blood flow to the kidneys.[681] It has also been shown that magnesium supplementation can help lower blood pressure, which is a known risk factor for kidney disease.[683] In the Healthy Aging in Neighborhoods of Diversity across the Life Span study they concluded that a lower dietary intake of magnesium was independently associated with a higher likelihood of rapid kidney function decline.[683]

As chronic kidney disease progresses, it leads to changes in mineral metabolism, with the severity worsening as the disease advances. It has been shown that among chronic kidney disease patients, low magnesium levels can increase the risk of progressing to end-stage renal disease and cardiovascular disease.[691] This may be due to magnesium's protective role in preventing arrhythmia and atherosclerosis in end stage renal disease patients.[681] Higher magnesium levels are advantageous for survival. Van Laecke et al. confirmed a link between low magnesium levels and an increased risk of death, as well as a faster decline in kidney function.[692] Magnesium may also improve clinical outcomes by preventing the progression of vascular calcification in chronic kidney disease.[693] Therefore it has been proposed that magnesium could be a valuable supplement in managing endothelial dysfunction and cardiovascular disease related to chronic kidney disease.[681]

Numerous studies indicate that correcting magnesium deficiency, or even supplementing magnesium when levels are not critically low, can enhance health and slow the progression of various diseases and pathological conditions. Individuals with chronic kidney disease commonly receive magnesium through oral supplements, dietary adjustments to include magnesium-rich foods, and adjustments in dialysate magnesium concentration for those undergoing hemodialysis or peritoneal dialysis.[684] Dietary magnesium primarily comes from green vegetables, nuts, seeds, and whole grains, but its bioavailability is greater in ripe fruits, fish, and meat. As we have mentioned in earlier chapters, it's important to note that the mineral content in plant and animal foods has significantly declined over the years due to modern farming practices, and processed foods generally have low magnesium content.[694] Magnesium carbonate is frequently prescribed for its ability to bind phosphate in cases of hyperphosphatemia (excess phosphate in the blood). The typical daily dosage of oral magnesium supplements varies widely across studies, ranging from 49 to 729 mg (2–30 mmol) of elemental magnesium per day.[684] In individuals with chronic kidney disease, magnesium supplementation can markedly slow the progression of vascular disease, showing notable benefits for arterial calcification, intima-media thickness, and calcification tendency. Additionally, magnesium positively influences mineral bone metabolism by improving serum calcium and parathyroid hormone levels.[684]

In summary, a low dietary intake of magnesium is significantly linked to a nearly two-fold increase in the likelihood of rapid kidney function decline. This association persists even after accounting for socio-demographic factors, kidney disease risk factors, baseline kidney function, and other dietary influences. This highlights the importance of adequate magnesium intake for individuals with chronic kidney disease.[683]

Magnesium and Kidney Stones

Kidney stones are hard deposits made of minerals and salts that form inside the kidneys, causing severe pain, blood in the urine, and possible urinary tract infections as they pass through the urinary system.[695] Kidney stones affect approximately 1–15% of the global population. They are often a recurrent condition, with a recurrence rate of 50% within 5–10 years and 75% within 20 years leading to significant socioeconomic and healthcare burdens in many countries.[696] Various risk factors contribute to the development of kidney stones, including genetic variations, lifestyle choices, environmental factors, and socioeconomic status.[697]

Magnesium, recognized for its ability to inhibit the formation of calcium oxalate crystals in the urine, was proposed as a prophylactic treatment for kidney stone disease as far back as the 17th and 18th centuries.[698] To date, only a limited number of human studies have explored the connection between serum magnesium levels and kidney stones. A case-control study revealed that patients with kidney stones (n = 100) had significantly lower serum magnesium levels compared to healthy controls (n = 100).[696] Previous human studies have indicated that individuals who develop calcium stones tend to have lower urinary magnesium levels compared to those who do not form stones.[699] These findings suggest that magnesium may play a protective and inhibitory role in preventing kidney stone formation.[699]

Calcium oxalate stones are the most prevalent type, making up the majority of all identified kidney stones.[699] Magnesium is believed to play a crucial role in the formation of kidney stones. In vitro studies have demonstrated that magnesium can inhibit several stages of kidney stone formation, including supersaturation, nucleation of calcium oxalate crystals, aggregation, and crystal growth. When bound in the urinary space, magnesium oxalate is 100 times more soluble than calcium oxalate. This significantly reduces the urinary saturation of calcium oxalate. Studies in an artificial urine environment at acidic pH have shown that magnesium not only binds with oxalate to reduce supersaturation but also decreases the time to reach supersaturation.[699] Once formed, calcium oxalate monohydrate crystals grow by adsorbing calcium and oxalate ions, promoting adhesion to kidney epithelial cells. Magnesium can slow down their growth and it competes with calcium oxalate monohydrate crystals, inhibiting their adhesion to kidney cells.[699] In addition to its direct impact on stone formation, magnesium can bind to oxalate in the gut, reducing its absorption. This further lowers the crystallization potential of calcium oxalate.[700, 701] In animal studies, low magnesium levels have been linked to the development of calcium oxalate monohydrate crystals, while dietary magnesium supplementation increased urinary magnesium and prevented the formation of calcium oxalate kidney stones.[699] Low urinary excretion of magnesium is recognized as a cause of increased calcium oxalate crystallization. Magnesium directly inhibits calcium oxalate crystallization in the urine, leading to increased urinary citrate excretion.[702] Low citrate levels in urine are a significant risk factor for kidney stone formation, as citrate inhibits calcium salt crystallization.[703] A leading cause of low citrate in the urine is lack of fruits or vegetables in the diet. This is one reason why it's important to balance the acid load of animal foods with fruits, vegetables or sodium/potassium bicarbonate or citrate.

In a study, researchers investigated the effects of feeding diets containing fructose, glucose, or starch, with or without added magnesium, on tissue levels of calcium in weanling rats. They found that animals fed a magnesium-deficient diet with fructose had the highest calcium content in their kidneys and hearts. The calcium content in the kidneys was particularly elevated, being 8 to 9 times greater than in other groups. These results show a synergistic effect between fructose and magnesium deficiency that significantly increases calcium levels in certain soft tissues, especially the kidneys, which increases the risk of kidney stones.[704]

In humans, those who form calcium stones typically have lower levels of urinary magnesium compared to non-stone formers.[699] In fact, over 25% of kidney stone patients have abnormally low urinary magnesium levels compared to urinary calcium levels.[705] A higher dietary magnesium intake is associated with a lower oxalate level in the urine of stone formers.[706] Magnesium supplementation appears to be as effective as diuretics in preventing kidney stone formation.[705] An interventional study by Kato et al. showed that magnesium supplementation reduced urinary oxalate levels.[707] Adding magnesium to drinking water could potentially also play a significant role in the primary prevention of kidney calcium stones.[705] Another study found that taking 391 mg of magnesium daily, as a mixed salt, magnesium/potassium citrate, reduced calcium stone recurrence by 90%. This was comparable to the effects of potassium citrate but with better tolerance for the digestive system.[708] Finally, in a study done by Johansson G. et al., they treated 55 patients with recurrent kidney calcium stones, who showed no signs of magnesium deficiency, with 500 mg of magnesium hydroxide daily for up to four years. Before treatment, the average stone rate was 0.8 stones per year per patient. The magnesium/calcium ratio in urine increased to levels seen in healthy individuals without stones. The average stone episode rate dropped from 0.8 to 0.08 stones per year, with 85% of treated patients remaining stone-free, compared to 59% of patients in the control group who continued forming stones. They concluded that magnesium treatment for kidney calcium stone disease is effective and has few side effects.[698]

In a study by Shringi, S. et al., utilizing data from the National Health and Nutrition Examination Survey (2011–2018), a large cohort of 19,271 individuals from the US population was examined. The study found a significant correlation between dietary magnesium intake and the likelihood of developing kidney stones. Their research showed that increased dietary magnesium intake is linked to a lower prevalence of kidney stone disease.[699] This is the most extensive population study to date investigating the impact of dietary magnesium intake on the risk of kidney stone formation, independent of other known risk factors.

Conclusion: Magnesium and Kidney Health

In summary, the value and benefits of magnesium in maintaining and improving kidney function are profound. This essential mineral offers significant advantages for individuals with chronic kidney disease by mitigating its progression through reducing inflammation, oxidative stress, and improving vascular function. Magnesium also protects against chronic kidney disease and plays a crucial role in preventing the formation of kidney calcium stones by increasing urinary magnesium excretion, improving the magnesium/calcium ratio, and boosting urinary citrate levels. Most importantly, magnesium supplementation is associated with minimal side effects, making it a safe and effective option for long-term kidney health management.

Incorporating magnesium into therapeutic regimens not only aids in the prevention and treatment of kidney stones and chronic kidney disease but also promotes overall kidney health, underscoring its importance as a vital nutrient in maintaining optimal kidney function.

Chapter 7: Magnesium and Diet

Diet plays a crucial role in our overall health, influencing various aspects of our well-being from physical vitality to mental clarity. What we eat directly impacts our body's ability to function optimally, affecting energy levels, immune response, and even mood. Unlike many factors affecting health that are beyond our control, such as genetics or environmental exposures, diet is one aspect we can manage actively. By making mindful choices about what we consume, we have the power to support our body's needs and promote long-term health.

The Standard American Diet (SAD), characterized by high intakes of processed foods, sugars, and unhealthy fats, has been linked to numerous health issues, including obesity, diabetes, heart disease, and certain cancers.[709] This diet typically lacks essential nutrients and is often devoid of the fresh fruits, vegetables, and lean proteins that are fundamental to a healthy diet. The negative impact of the Standard American Diet on public health is profound, highlighting the urgent need for dietary reform to address the rising prevalence of diet-related diseases.[709]

Despite modern agricultural practices leading to a decrease in the nutrient density of our foods, our diet remains a key avenue for nourishing the body. Soil depletion, use of chemical fertilizers, and other farming techniques have contributed to lower levels of vitamins and minerals in produce.[710-712] Nevertheless, a well-balanced diet, rich in a variety of whole foods, continues to be essential for maintaining health. By prioritizing nutrient-dense foods and minimizing processed food consumption, we can provide our bodies with the necessary building blocks for optimal health.

In this chapter, we will explore the specific role of diet in managing magnesium levels in the body. Our dietary choices can significantly influence magnesium intake and absorption, which in turn affects overall health. We will examine how different foods and dietary patterns can either enhance or hinder magnesium levels in the body. Finally, we will provide practical guidance for incorporating magnesium-rich foods into the diet to support optimal health.

Refined Carbohydrates and Sugar Deplete Magnesium Levels

Refined carbohydrates and refined sugars are prevalent in our modern diet, especially in North America, where convenience and taste often take precedence over nutritional value. Refined carbohydrates are those that have been processed to remove the bran and germ from whole grains, resulting in a finer texture and longer shelf life but stripping away fiber, vitamins, and minerals. Common examples include white flour, white rice, and many types of bread and pastries. Similarly, refined sugars are processed to remove molasses and impurities from natural sources like sugar cane and sugar beets, resulting in products like white sugar, high-fructose corn syrup, and other sweeteners found in a vast array of foods.

Historically, sugar consumption included beneficial plant antioxidants (polyphenols), fiber, vitamins, and minerals. The fiber in these whole foods reduced sugar absorption and slowed its release into the bloodstream, preventing blood sugar spikes and subsequent crashes that lead to more sugar cravings. This fiber would also produce healthy short-chain fatty acids in the colon, improving insulin sensitivity and glucose tolerance, allowing the body to handle sugar without harm.[713] Additionally, foraging for food, which often involved physical activity, further improved our ancestors' insulin sensitivity and glucose tolerance, priming their bodies for sugar consumption.

In contrast, modern sugar consumption is vastly different. Sugar is now hidden in nearly 75% of all packaged foods, requires no physical effort to obtain, and provides no nutritional value. Instead, refined sugars and carbohydrates act as "anti-nutrients," depleting the body of essential nutrients needed to metabolize them. Among the nutrients depleted by refined sugar and carbohydrates is magnesium, a crucial mineral for our health.[714]

Since 1940, there has been a significant decline in the micronutrient density of foods.[711] The reduction in magnesium during food processing and refining is particularly significant. For example, white flour loses 82% of its magnesium, polished rice loses 83%, starch loses 97%, and white sugar loses 99%.[17] Refined carbohydrates and added sugars lack magnesium yet demand magnesium for their metabolism in the body. Consequently, the more refined carbohydrates and sugars one consumes, the more depleted one's magnesium levels become.[715]

Since 1840, the magnesium content of wheat dropped 33%.[716] This decline is potentially due to factors such as acidic soil, yield dilution, and unbalanced fertilization practices. High levels of nitrogen, phosphorus, and potassium in the soil can hinder magnesium absorption in plants.[717] A review paper concluded that magnesium deficiency in plants is becoming a more serious issue due to the advancement of industry and agriculture, as well as the growing human population.[717] Processed foods, fats, refined flour, and sugars lack magnesium, making the Western diet prone to magnesium deficiency.[1]

Magnesium acts as a crucial second messenger in insulin signaling, while insulin itself regulates the accumulation of magnesium within cells. Low intracellular magnesium levels may contribute to the impaired insulin response seen in Type 2 diabetes.[603] This connection explains how refined carbohydrates and sugars can lead to magnesium deficiency by promoting insulin resistance. In diabetes, decreased magnesium within cells is believed to result from both increased urinary losses and insulin resistance.[603] This was covered in detail in chapter 5.

Ten ways sugar and refined carbohydrates deplete your body of magnesium.

1. **Lack of Magnesium Content:** Refined carbohydrates and added sugars provide little to no magnesium, yet the enzymes needed to metabolize glucose and fructose require magnesium for their function.[714]

2. **Vitamin-B6 Depletion**: Metabolizing sugar depletes the body of vitamin-B6[718], which is essential for magnesium absorption and transport into cells.[143, 144]

3. **Insulin Resistance:** Sugar and refined carbohydrate consumption can lead to insulin resistance[82, 83], which impairs magnesium transport into cells[84], leading to intracellular magnesium deficiency.

4. **Urinary Magnesium Loss**: Elevated blood sugar and insulin levels result in magnesium being excreted out the urine.[65, 113]

5. **Oxidative Stress:** Increased oxidative stress from sugar and refined carbohydrate intake requires greater use of antioxidant enzymes that rely partially on magnesium for their function.[719-721]

6. **Bone Magnesium Depletion:** Hyperglycemia-induced lactic acid production from osteoclasts may strip magnesium salts from bones.[722]

7. **Diarrhea-Induced Loss:** Fructose, in particular, can cause diarrhea, leading to magnesium loss in the feces.[723, 724]

8. **Increased Aldosterone Levels:** Elevated leptin levels/leptin resistance from sugar consumption increase aldosterone, which can lead to magnesium loss through urine.[725, 726]

9. **Salt Deficiency:** Overconsuming sugar and refined carbohydrates can damage the intestinal cells, kidney cells and cause osmotic diuresis leading to decreased salt absorption and salt wasting out the urine.[727] Sodium deficiency can then lead to:[90, 131, 728, 729]

    a. Stripping of magnesium from bones (to get the sodium from the bones that the body demands but magnesium and calcium are also stripped simultaneously)

    b. Increased magnesium loss in sweat as the body conserves sodium

    c. Elevated aldosterone, which expels magnesium in urine

10. **Phosphoric Acid in Soft Drinks:** Soft drinks containing phosphoric acid increase the need for magnesium as phosphates bind to magnesium in the intestinal tract, reducing its absorption.[1, 730]

Glucose and refined carbohydrates can also affect bone health. As mentioned, a diet high in refined sugar can lead to hyperinsulinemia, causing calcium and magnesium to be excreted in the urine due to insulin's inhibition of renal tubular reabsorption of calcium and magnesium.[731, 732] A deficiency in calcium and magnesium can reduce bone formation and mineralization[733], leading to poor bone crystallization and an increased risk of osteoporosis.[35] Excessive sugar intake can significantly increase the body's need for magnesium. In a study involving young men, magnesium excretion in the urine significantly increased (in some individuals more than doubling) after consuming 100 grams of glucose.[734]

Dietary Factors Affecting Magnesium Status

Dietary factors play a crucial role in determining magnesium status, influencing how much magnesium our bodies can absorb, retain, and utilize effectively. Many seemingly healthy individuals are at risk of insufficient magnesium intake due to the reduced presence of magnesium in the modern Western diet. This is largely attributed to factors such as the widespread use of demineralized water, consumption of processed foods, and agricultural practices that rely on magnesium-deficient soil.[715]

Although magnesium intake has been gradually declining since the start of the century, the demand for this mineral has sharply increased due to higher consumption of certain nutrients, particularly vitamin D, calcium and phosphorus. A primary source of phosphorus is soft drinks containing phosphoric acid, and the consumption of these beverages has significantly risen over the past 25 years.

Higher intakes of calcium and phosphorus can elevate the body's magnesium requirements, potentially exacerbating or leading to magnesium deficiency.[735-737] Dairy products, particularly cheese, exhibit a notably high phosphorus-to-magnesium ratio. For instance, cheddar cheese has a phosphorus-to-magnesium ratio of approximately 18 and a calcium-to-magnesium ratio of around 26.[738] Some experts suggest that the ideal dietary calcium-to-magnesium ratio is around 2:1.[20]

The dietary magnesium needed to maintain a positive balance varies based on numerous factors, including patient population, diet, and lifestyle choices. For example, magnesium balance tends to decrease when calcium intake exceeds 10 mg per kg per day. [26] This isn't to say that you shouldn't consume more than 10 mg/kg/day of calcium, it just means that magnesium needs may increase once the calcium intake is above that amount. Therefore, the minimum required magnesium intake to achieve a positive balance is not universal. Magnesium interacts with several other nutrients, and its requirement is influenced not only by their levels but also by their forms. The typical American diet is low in calcium and magnesium but high in protein and phosphorus. Excessive intake of calcium, phosphorus, and vitamin D can also lead to increased magnesium loss, further raising magnesium requirements.

From 1932 to 1939, the phosphate-to-calcium ratio in the USA was approximately 1.2 to 1. However, for those who replaced milk with soda, this ratio increased to 4 to 1. Other data suggests that the current phosphate-to-calcium ratio is around 1.5:1.[1] The most significant change since the early 1900s has been a substantial reduction in magnesium intake, dropping from about 500 mg/day to 175-225 mg/day.[739] Consequently, the calcium-to-magnesium ratio has risen from roughly 2:1 to 5:1, and the phosphate-to-magnesium ratio has increased from 1.2:1 to about 7:1.[1] The surge in dietary phosphate primarily comes from phosphate additives in various foods, particularly processed meats, and from phosphoric acid found in soft drinks.

One group of researchers concluded that the prevalence and incidence of Type 2 diabetes in the United States increased sharply between 1994 and 2001 as the calcium-to-magnesium intake ratio from food rose from below 3.0 to above 3.0.[24] Another study found a 3.25-fold increased risk of diabetes when plasma magnesium levels were below 0.863 mmol/L, even though 0.75 mmol/L is considered a "normal" level.[22] As we have mentioned before, this suggests that patients with diabetes are often magnesium-deficient, and that magnesium deficiency likely increases the risk of developing diabetes.

Dietary aluminum can contribute to magnesium deficiency by significantly reducing magnesium absorption by approximately five-fold and decreasing magnesium retention by 41%, which in turn lowers magnesium levels in bones.[740] Given the widespread presence of aluminum in modern society, including in cookware, deodorants, medications, over the counter supplements, baking powder, and baked goods, it could be a major factor in magnesium deficiency. Lastly, a diet deficient in vitamin B6 can lead to a negative magnesium balance by increasing magnesium excretion.[143]

The Role of Dietary Calcium in Regulating Magnesium Balance

The interplay between dietary calcium and magnesium balance is complex and significant, as calcium intake can directly impact magnesium levels and overall mineral equilibrium in the body.

In a series of magnesium balance studies conducted by Seelig around 60 years ago, it was observed that men with magnesium intakes at or above the recommended dietary allowance (6 mg per kg per day) maintained their magnesium balance even when dietary calcium levels were increased to high amounts.[6] This finding aligns with more recent research on the topic.[24]

In men with relatively low magnesium intakes, high calcium intake was shown to disrupt magnesium balance.[6] Interestingly, a low calcium intake also negatively affected magnesium availability in this group. If similar effects are observed in women, it suggests that high supplemental calcium intake could impair magnesium balance in a significant portion of the population with low magnesium levels, reflecting diets rich in "empty calorie" foods. However, consuming calcium-rich natural foods may not have the same negative impact, as these foods also provide magnesium. For instance, a cup of milk can contribute up to 10% of the daily magnesium requirement. Additional balance studies are necessary to verify Seelig's observation that high calcium intake may disrupt magnesium balance when magnesium levels are relatively low.[6]

Calcium and magnesium are not believed to share common transport proteins in the intestinal mucosa or renal tubular epithelium[741, 742], so the exact mechanism behind their antagonistic interaction remains unclear. Brink and colleagues have demonstrated that this effect is dependent on a sufficiently high intake of phosphate.[730] Their research shows that increased calcium intake can reduce the solubility of dietary magnesium in the ileum by forming insoluble calcium/magnesium/phosphate complexes. This interaction is most pronounced when the dietary phosphate-to-magnesium ratio is relatively high. Brink et al. suggest that since this ratio is higher in rat diets compared to human diets, high calcium intake may not significantly impact magnesium balance in most clinical studies involving humans.[730] However, individuals consuming overly processed diets low in magnesium, yet high in bioavailable phosphate from animal products and additives, might experience further disruption of magnesium status due to high supplemental calcium intake.[743]

It has been proposed that high calcium intake could suppress parathyroid hormone and/or calcitriol levels, potentially reducing the efficiency of magnesium absorption.[744] Several studies in both humans and rats suggest that administering calcitriol (the active form of vitamin D) can enhance magnesium absorption in the intestines, with human studies showing increased jejunal absorption of magnesium.[745-748] Thus, both a lack of vitamin D, or too much vitamin D, can contribute to magnesium deficiency.[1]

The Impact of Prolonged Fasting on Magnesium Levels

Prolonged fasting involves abstaining from food for an extended period, typically exceeding 24 hours. This practice is often undertaken for various reasons, including medical, religious, or wellness purposes. From a medical standpoint, prolonged fasting can be used as a therapeutic intervention for managing certain health conditions, such as obesity, metabolic syndrome, or autoimmune disorders.[749] In religious or spiritual contexts, fasting serves as a form of purification and spiritual discipline.[750] Additionally, some individuals turn to prolonged fasting for potential benefits like improved mental clarity, enhanced metabolic health, or detoxification.[751] It's essential to approach prolonged fasting with caution and understanding, as it can have significant impacts on the body's nutritional status and overall health.

One such impact is magnesium. During fasting, the body shifts its primary energy source from carbohydrates to fatty acids and amino acids. While serum mineral levels stay normal, many intracellular minerals (magnesium included) become significantly depleted during this time.[752] Prolonged fasting is linked to ongoing magnesium loss, with some individuals experiencing a deficit of up to 20% of their total body magnesium after two months.[122] Most of this loss occurs through the kidneys, although the intestines may also contribute in certain cases. Muscle magnesium levels may drop by 20% after fasting, but the overall magnesium deficit often exceeds what would be expected from lean tissue loss alone. Despite muscle depletion, plasma magnesium levels generally remain stable. Persistent magnesium loss during fasting may be influenced by the body's increased acid load and lack of insulin. Magnesium excretion tends to increase with the severity of acidosis, but glucose consumption can help reduce magnesium loss.[122]

In a study conducted by Stewart and Fleming, 19 obese patients underwent an 18-day fast.[753] Among those who received no supplements or only calcium or sodium supplements, plasma magnesium levels decreased by 9% to 25%. However, patients who were given magnesium supplements did not experience this decline. Erythrocyte magnesium levels remained stable across all groups, but erythrocyte potassium levels dropped by 5% to 9% in patients with reduced plasma magnesium levels and stayed unchanged in those receiving magnesium supplements.[753] In another study by the same researchers, a 27-year-old patient who fasted for 382 days experienced a consistent decrease in plasma magnesium concentrations, beginning from the first month onward.[754] Finally, in healthy individuals on a magnesium-deficient diet, the loss of magnesium through urine and feces is usually low, around 1 mEq/day. However, in fasting obese men urinary magnesium excretion was found to be four to five times higher.[122]

Impact of Various Dietary Patterns and Nutrients on Magnesium Levels

There are countless dietary approaches available today, each with its unique emphasis, whether it's high-protein, high-fat, low-carb, or plant-based. These diets are not just trends but often serve specific therapeutic purposes, tailored to address various health issues. For instance, a high-protein diet might be used to support muscle growth or weight loss, while a ketogenic diet could be employed to manage epilepsy or metabolic disorders. The choice of diet often depends on the individual's health needs, goals, and how their body responds to different nutrients. Here we will explore how different dietary patterns influence magnesium levels.

Many metabolic balance studies reveal that certain nutrients and stress conditions can increase magnesium requirements. Dietary surveys also show that many self-selected diets provide only 200-250 mg of magnesium per day, falling short of the recommended 310-420 mg per day for adults.[1] The intake of key nutrients that elevate magnesium requirements, such as calcium, phosphate, and vitamin D, has significantly increased.

Animal studies indicate that high ratios of calcium/magnesium, phosphate/magnesium, and excess vitamin D can lead to magnesium deficiency.[1]

Sufficient protein intake is essential for optimal magnesium retention. Studies have shown that when protein intake was increased from low to normal levels in young boys, adolescent boys, girls, and women on diets low in magnesium, their magnesium retention improved. Diets providing adequate magnesium for growth and development (around 10-16 mg/kg/day) led to positive magnesium balances, regardless of protein intake. Additionally, high magnesium intake has been found to enhance nitrogen balance in individuals consuming a high-protein diet.[755] Protein loading, such as consuming large amounts of whey protein for example, alongside a normal diet, can lead to magnesium loss through urine due to the acid load. A low magnesium-to-protein ratio may put individuals at risk of magnesium depletion. Increasing this ratio can improve both magnesium and nitrogen balance, emphasizing the need for sufficient magnesium intake to support optimal health.[755]

In a paper by S. Johnson, he points out that the modern American diet, characterized by hamburgers, French fries, coffee, and sodas, is deficient in magnesium and high in saturated fats, which further inhibits the absorption of magnesium.[98] In addition, it has been shown that elevated fat levels in the intestines, whether from consuming fatty foods or due to conditions like steatorrhea or short bowel syndrome, can hinder magnesium absorption.[755] This occurs because fat combines with magnesium and other divalent cations to form soaps, which the body cannot absorb.[755] This indicates that a low-carbohydrate, high-fat diet might have drawbacks if it is not complemented by a sufficient intake of magnesium or if magnesium is not spaced from high fat intakes. Balancing such a diet with magnesium-rich foods or supplements could be crucial to mitigate potential negative effects.

Cardioprotective diets typically emphasize reduced intake of total and saturated fats, a balanced supply of monounsaturated fats and omega-3 fatty acids, moderate alcohol consumption, and increased consumption of whole grains, fruits, vegetables, fish, and low-fat dairy. Magnesium is especially important in these diets due to the common occurrence of chronic magnesium deficiency, which is a cardiovascular risk factor.

Additionally, these diets naturally tend to be high in magnesium, further supporting heart health.[756]

Alcohol has long been a prevalent and socially accepted part of cultures worldwide, yet its widespread use also brings complex challenges and health implications. Excessive alcohol consumption, whether with or without food, raises magnesium requirements, as it increases urinary magnesium loss.[755] Poor diet and excessive alcohol use are major contributors to severe magnesium depletion, a condition that has been clinically recognized as a serious health issue.

Thiamine, or vitamin B1, is essential for energy metabolism and plays a critical role in converting carbohydrates into energy the body can use. It supports proper nerve function, muscle contraction, and the production of neurotransmitters, making it vital for maintaining overall physical and mental well-being.[757] Thiamine requires magnesium to be converted into its active form called thiamine pyrophosphate, which is crucial for many functions in the body. Without enough magnesium, thiamine cannot work effectively, leading to symptoms of thiamine deficiency even if the body has sufficient amounts. This can result in low gastric acid levels, increasing the risk of gastrointestinal infections and impairing digestion, as well as causing damage to the hypothalamus, which may lead to neurological issues like confusion, delusions, and Wernicke's encephalopathy.[98] Foods high in thiamine include whole grains like brown rice and oatmeal, legumes such as lentils and black beans, nuts and seeds like sunflower seeds and macadamia nuts, pork, fish such as tuna and trout, fortified cereals, eggs, and organ meats like liver and kidneys.[757] However, the more carbohydrates consumed, the more magnesium is needed by the body (and the same goes for thiamine). Thus, just because a food contains high amounts of thiamine or magnesium, does not necessarily mean it contributes well to the thiamine/magnesium status of the body. Typically, higher fiber, higher carbohydrate foods, contribute less to the magnesium status of the body, even though they tend to be the highest magnesium sources because fiber lowers the absorption of magnesium and carbohydrates increase magnesium need. However, this depends on the type of fiber.

Inulin, a prebiotic that promotes beneficial gut bacteria, has been shown to nearly double magnesium absorption in the large intestine. On the other hand, large amounts of psyllium seed husks significantly decreases magnesium absorption, and gum arabic raises both intestinal and renal excretion of magnesium, making them less ideal for those needing magnesium.[758] One study examined whether the consumption of fructo-oligosaccharides (FOS) improved mineral absorption. What they found was that after 36 days of consuming short-chain fructo-oligosaccharides (sc-FOS) (foods that contain these are bananas, asparagus and Jerusalem artichoke), magnesium absorption increased by 18%.[759]

Finally, proper hydration is crucial for maintaining optimal mineral balance in the body. When water intake is insufficient, the body compensates by excreting more magnesium to increase urine salinity, similar to the effects of consuming too much sodium.[98]

Magnesium Rich Foods

Although modern agricultural practices have led to a decline in the magnesium content of our soils, which can affect the nutrient levels in our food[75], we can still obtain adequate amounts of this vital mineral through a well-balanced diet. By focusing on diverse and nutrient-rich dietary choices, individuals can help to support their magnesium needs and overall health.

Around 65% of the American population consumes a diet that falls short of meeting adequate magnesium levels. Data from the 2005–2006 National Health and Nutrition Examination Survey indicated that magnesium intake is below the Estimated Average Requirement across all age groups, with adult men aged 71 and older, as well as adolescent women, being particularly prone to insufficient intake.[760] Over the past 50 years, there has been a notable decline in magnesium intake among the U.S. population. This decrease is attributed to a reduction in the consumption of magnesium-rich foods, while the intake of magnesium-poor foods has increased.

Magnesium is found abundantly in both plant and animal foods. Key sources include spinach, legumes, nuts, seeds, whole grains, meat, seafood, bananas and avocados. Food processing methods, such as refining grains that strip away the nutrient-rich germ and bran, can significantly reduce the magnesium content.[757] It is important to note that some of these "high magnesium foods", like spinach (high in oxalates), legumes (high in carbohydrates) and nuts, seeds and whole grains (high in phytate and fiber) have a

182

lower bioavailability/contribution of magnesium to the body compared to magnesium found in meat, seafood or avocados for example. Additionally, many people do not tolerate nuts, seeds, grains, or spinach. Thus, if you consume mostly animal foods and simply supplement with extra magnesium, that may be a better strategy for many people, rather than trying to consume these "high magnesium foods" that many people don't tolerate.

High Magnesium Content Foods (Adapted from NIH)[757]

Food	Milligrams (Mg) per serving	Percent Daily Value
Pumpkin seeds, 1 ounce	156	37
Chia seeds, 1 ounce	111	26
Almonds, 1 ounce	80	19
Spinach, ½ cup	78	19
Cashews, 1 ounce	74	18
Dark Chocolate, 1 ounce[761]	64	15
Peanuts, ¼ cup	63	15
Soy milk, 1 cup	61	15
Black beans ½ cup	60	14
Edamame, ½ cup	50	12
Peanut Butter, 2 tbsp.	49	12
Potato, baked, 3.5 ounces	43	10
Rice, brown ½ cup	42	10

Yogurt, plain, 8 ounces	42	10
Breakfast cereals, fortified with 10% of the DV for magnesium, 1 serving	42	10
Oatmeal, Instant, 1 packet	36	9
Kidney beans, ½ cup	35	8
Banana, 1 medium	32	8
Salmon, Atlantic, 3 ounces	26	6
Milk, 1 cup	24-27	6
Halibut, 3 ounces	24	6
Raisins, ½ cup	23	5
Bread, whole wheat, 1 slice	23	5
Avocado, ½ cup	22	5
Chicken breast, 3 ounces	22	5
Beef, ground, 90% lean, 3 ounces	20	5
Broccoli, ½ cup	12	3
Rice, white, ½ cup	10	2
Apple, 1 medium	9	2
Carrot, 1 medium	7	2

Intake Recommendations

The World Health Organization (WHO), Food and Agriculture Organization (FAO), American National Academy of Medicine (NAM), and European Food Safety Agency (EFSA) have all provided intake recommendations for magnesium and other nutrients.[715]

These values, which differ based on sex and age, help guide diet planning for individuals and the general population.[715] They include:

- **Recommended Dietary Allowances (RDAs)** have been updated and renamed as **Dietary Reference Intakes (DRIs)**. This is the recommended daily nutrient intake levels to meet the needs of most healthy people.[715]

- **Population Reference Intakes (PRIs):** The nutrient level adequate for most people in a population.

- **Average Requirements (ARs):** The intake level sufficient for 50% of healthy individuals, used for assessing and planning diets.

- **Adequate Intake (AI):** The assumed intake level needed to ensure nutritional adequacy.

- **Tolerable Upper Intake Level (UL):** The maximum daily intake considered safe without adverse health effects for the population.

Magnesium Intake Recommendations[715]

Life Stage	PRI (mg)	AR (mg)	UL (mg)	RDA-DRI (mg)	DRV-AI (mg)
Birth to 6 months	-	-	Nd	30	-
Infants 7-12 months	80	Nd	Nd	75	80

Children 1-3 years	80	65	250	80	170
Children 4-6 years	100	85	250	130	230
Children 7-10 years	150	130	250	240	230
Teen boys 11-18 years	240	170-200	250	410	300
Teen girls 11-18 years	240	170-200	250	360	250
Men	240	170	250	400-420	350
Women	240	170	250	310-320	300
Pregnant	240	170	250	350-400	300
Breastfeeding	240	170	250	310-360	300

Considering the data showing that approximately 60% of adults have insufficient magnesium intake, it's clear that subclinical magnesium deficiency is a prevalent issue in the Western population.[1] Given magnesium's crucial role in numerous bodily functions and its potential preventive benefits against various health conditions, it is essential to prioritize adequate magnesium intake. Incorporating magnesium-rich, non-refined foods into your diet, such as meat, seafood, and certain fruits like avocados and bananas, and if tolerated, leafy greens, nuts, seeds, and whole grains, is a simple and cost-effective way to boost your magnesium levels.

Additionally, considering magnesium supplementation can be a beneficial strategy for those who struggle to meet their daily needs through diet alone. We will be covering supplementation in the next chapter. Ultimately, by paying closer attention to dietary magnesium intake, we can take a proactive step toward better health and well-being.

Chapter 8: Magnesium Supplementation: Forms, Absorption, and Efficacy

As we have mentioned many times, magnesium is the cornerstone of our well-being. It is involved in countless bodily functions that keep us thriving. Yet, despite its importance, magnesium deficiency remains alarmingly common. Throughout this book, we have explored how modern lifestyles and dietary habits often fall short in providing adequate magnesium, leading to a range of health challenges. For many, the gap between what we need and what we consume has become too wide, making magnesium supplementation not just beneficial, but essential.

But not all magnesium supplements are created equal. The market is flooded with different forms of magnesium, each with distinct strengths, weaknesses, and specific uses. From highly absorbable forms to those that the body absorbs less effectively, each form of magnesium has its own unique characteristics. It is important to realize that the choice of supplement can dramatically affect how well the body absorbs and utilizes this vital mineral. Understanding the nuances of each form is key to selecting the right magnesium supplement that meets individual needs.

In this final chapter, we will examine the most common magnesium supplements and review research on the various forms. The aim is to provide the knowledge necessary to make an informed decision, ensuring that the supplementation process is both effective and tailored to individual needs. With this information, selecting the magnesium supplement that best addresses health concerns will be easier, helping to bridge the gap in magnesium deficiency and unlock the full benefits of this essential mineral.

Finally, it is recommended to always work with a healthcare practitioner when starting any new supplement to ensure safety and effectiveness. While dosages from studies and research papers will be referenced, this information is not intended as medical advice.

The Recommended Dietary Allowance

The Recommended Dietary Allowance (RDA) for magnesium in adults ranges from 310 to 420 mg per day. For most adult women the RDA ranges from 310-360 mg, whereas for adult men it ranges from 410-420 mg per day. This represents the average daily intake level sufficient to meet the nutrient needs of nearly all (97 to 98 percent) healthy individuals within a specific life stage and gender group.[762] However, there are situations where this baseline may be insufficient. Individuals with gastrointestinal disorders that impair magnesium absorption, those taking medications that deplete magnesium, or those whose diets are high in processed foods and low in magnesium-rich options may need to increase their magnesium intake.[552] Additionally, those engaged in intense physical activity or under significant stress may also need increased magnesium levels to meet their body's demands.[552] While the recommended dietary allowance serves as a helpful guideline, individual factors should be considered, and magnesium intake adjusted accordingly.

Magnesium and Amino Acids

Some forms of magnesium are combined with amino acids to enhance stability and absorption in the body. When magnesium combines with amino acids, the resulting compounds are more bioavailable and give higher magnesium levels in the bloodstream compared to other magnesium compounds. These magnesium–amino acid compounds are absorbed more effectively through dipeptide channels in the gut, which are more abundant than ion channels, enhancing their absorption. The stability of these bonds also helps protect magnesium from chemical reactions that could hinder absorption. Differences in how these compounds are absorbed and used by the body may depend on the specific amino acids involved.[763]

Magnesium Forms

In the following section, we will dive into the different forms of magnesium that are being sold as supplements. It is important to recognize that while there are various forms of magnesium, each tailored to address specific health concerns, many of these forms also share overlapping benefits.

Magnesium Hydroxide

Magnesium dihydroxide, commonly known as magnesium hydroxide, is an inorganic compound where the magnesium atom is bound to two hydroxide groups. Naturally occurring as the mineral brucite, magnesium hydroxide serves multiple purposes.[764] In water, it forms a suspension known as milk of magnesia, which has been widely used for many years as both an antacid and a laxative.[765] It is available in both oral liquid suspension and chewable tablet forms. Magnesium hydroxide can also be applied topically as a deodorant or for relieving canker sores (aphthous ulcers).[764]

Magnesium hydroxide acts as an antacid in low doses.[764] It works through a simple neutralization process. Hydroxide ions from magnesium combine with the acidic hydronium ions produced by the stomach's parietal cells resulting in the formation of water.[766] This reaction not only neutralizes stomach acid but also increases the pH of the stomach contents, offering relief from the burning sensation commonly associated with heartburn and indigestion.[766] At doses of 400 mg to 1,200 mg it functions as an antacid but in higher doses it functions as a laxative.[764, 767] As a laxative, magnesium hydroxide is typically administered as a suspension at a concentration ranging from 800-2,400 mg per 10 milliliters at a dose of 2,400 to 4,800 mg at once or in divided doses (and typically not to exceed 4,800 mg total per day).[767] Its effectiveness stems from several mechanisms. The magnesium ions are poorly absorbed in the intestinal tract, leading to an osmotic effect that draws water into the intestines. This increase in water content softens the stool and boosts its volume, naturally stimulating intestinal motility. Additionally, magnesium ions trigger the release of cholecystokinin (CCK), which further promotes water and electrolyte accumulation in the intestines, enhancing motility.[768, 769]

Magnesium hydroxide can cause side effects, though they are typically mild and manageable. Common side effects include diarrhea, which is expected due to its laxative properties and it can sometimes lead to dehydration and electrolyte imbalances, especially with high doses and prolonged use. Other potential side effects, such as abdominal cramping, nausea, and vomiting, are usually mild and tend to resolve as the body adjusts.[770]

Magnesium hydroxide should be used with caution in certain individuals. Those with kidney disease should avoid it without medical supervision.[771] Magnesium hydroxide contains a relatively high percentage of elemental magnesium but has low solubility in water[762], which suggests poor absorption. It is essential to adhere to the dosage instructions provided on the packaging or by a healthcare professional.

Magnesium Oxide

Magnesium oxide was introduced to East Asia in the 19th century by German physician P.F.B. Siebold, who brought it to Japan. Since then, it has become a widely used laxative in countries like Japan, China, and Taiwan.[772] Magnesium oxide is cost-effective, and its small molecular size allows for a high concentration of elemental magnesium to be delivered without taking up much space in a tablet or a capsule.

Magnesium oxide is an osmotic laxative.[772] It has been recommended as a first-line treatment in clinical practice guidelines for chronic constipation due to its high safety profile and minimal risk of serious adverse events.[773] Magnesium oxide works by converting into magnesium chloride in the acidic environment of the stomach. In the duodenum, magnesium chloride is further converted into magnesium bicarbonate by sodium hydrogen carbonate from pancreatic secretions, and eventually into magnesium carbonate. These compounds increase the osmotic pressure within the intestinal lumen, drawing water into the intestines, which raises the water content and volume of the stool. Additionally, the increased stool volume stimulates the intestinal wall and enhances intestinal propulsive motor activity.[772]

Mori S et al. conducted a randomized, double-blind, placebo-controlled study comparing magnesium oxide with a placebo.[774] The study demonstrated the effectiveness of magnesium oxide in treating chronic constipation. Magnesium oxide significantly improved overall symptoms, spontaneous bowel movements, stool form, colonic transit time, abdominal discomfort, and quality of life. Patients treated with magnesium oxide had a 70.6% response rate for overall symptom improvement, compared to just 25.0% in the placebo group.[774]

Magnesium oxide has traditionally been regarded as a poor source of magnesium due to its insolubility in water and the pH conditions in the small intestine, leading to a bioavailability of 4%.[775] Due to the low bioavailability, many subjects report frequent digestive upset (loose bowel movements, nausea, gastrointestinal distress), especially at high doses.[776]

Magnesium Chloride

Magnesium chloride is an inorganic compound composed of one magnesium ion and two chloride ions. It is highly soluble in water. Magnesium chloride is primarily obtained from brine or seawater, with rich sources found in the Great Salt Lake in North America and the Dead Sea in the Jordan Valley.[764]

Research studies have demonstrated positive clinical outcomes with magnesium chloride. For instance, a randomized, double-blind, placebo-controlled study by Rodriguez-Moran and Guerrero-Romero found that magnesium chloride supplementation improved the metabolic profile and blood pressure in overweight individuals.[777] Similarly, another study looked at whether oral magnesium supplementation influenced serum levels of high-sensitivity C-reactive protein (hsCRP) in healthy subjects with prediabetes and hypomagnesemia. C-reactive protein is a marker of inflammation. The study concluded that magnesium chloride reduced C-reactive protein levels.[778] Tarelton et al. demonstrated that a 6-week regimen of magnesium chloride significantly improved both depression and anxiety symptoms.[417] Daily intake of 248 mg of elemental magnesium chloride resulted in a statistically and clinically significant result. Depression scores improved by an average of 6 points on the PHQ-9 and anxiety scores improved by over 4 points on the GAD-7.[417]

Magnesium chloride is available as a supplement that can be taken orally to increase magnesium levels in the body or applied topically to provide local skeletal muscle effects. The bioavailability of magnesium chloride is good.[776] Soluble forms of magnesium are more readily absorbed in the gastrointestinal tract compared to less soluble forms. Magnesium chloride, being a soluble form of magnesium, is absorbed in the gastrointestinal tract.[715] Its effects are dose-dependent: while it is generally well-tolerated at moderate doses, higher doses may induce a laxative effect, potentially causing diarrhea or gastrointestinal discomfort.[776]

In recent years there has been a growing popularity of transdermal applications, such as magnesium sprays, flakes, and salt baths. There has been debate around transdermal magnesium being superior to oral supplements, citing better absorption and fewer side effects since it bypasses the gastrointestinal tract. Current studies raise concerns about the effectiveness of transdermal magnesium and at this point lacks scientific validation.[779] It is particularly alarming if reliance on this method leads to unsuccessful treatment outcomes. Future research needs to explore the impact of transdermal magnesium on a larger population, using higher concentrations and longer application periods, to determine if it can significantly improve magnesium levels by potentially bypassing the gastrointestinal tract. However, until more conclusive evidence is available, we cannot recommend the use of transdermal magnesium for improving magnesium status of the body. There may be some local benefits to the skin and/or muscle with the use of topical magnesium.

Magnesium Citrate

Magnesium citrate is commonly used and has been studied for numerous health conditions. It is a form of magnesium that is bound to citric acid and has been described as a laxative.[780] Magnesium citrate dissolves easily in water, making it suitable for use in powder, capsule, or liquid form.

Magnesium citrate's mechanism of action involves attracting water through osmosis. When it reaches the intestine, it draws in sufficient water to stimulate motility and induce defecation. This makes it effective for treating occasional constipation and irregularity issues.[781] When using magnesium citrate for regularity and constipation, it is most effective when taken on an empty stomach, followed by a full glass of water to enhance absorption and counteract water loss.[781]

A study looked at how different organic magnesium compounds transition into tissues at various doses. They found that tissue magnesium levels increased in a dose-dependent manner in the magnesium citrate groups which implies that magnesium citrate is effective at high doses.[763] This was seen in the following study. Researchers conducted a double-blind, randomized, placebo-controlled study to assess the preventive effects of 600 mg/day of oral magnesium citrate in patients with migraines without aura.[782] Over a 3-month treatment period, clinical assessments, visual evoked potentials, and brain SPECT imaging revealed that magnesium supplementation led to reductions in both the frequency and severity of migraine attacks. It was concluded that magnesium citrate may be an effective option for migraine prophylaxis, likely working through both vascular and neurogenic mechanisms.[782]

Research suggests that magnesium citrate may benefit older adults with insomnia. Randomized control trials indicate that oral magnesium citrate supplements can improve sleep parameters, including sleep onset latency and total sleep time, offering potential relief for insomnia symptoms.[783] In a study of adults over the age of 51 with poor sleep quality, a daily supplement of 320 mg of magnesium citrate significantly improved sleep quality and disturbances as measured by the Pittsburgh Sleep Quality Index (PSQI).[354]

In a very recent open-label pilot study involving adults with primary restless legs syndrome, daily administration of 200 mg of magnesium citrate for 8 weeks led to significant improvements.[784] Participants experienced a notable reduction in Restless Legs Syndrome symptom scores and improved quality of life without significant changes in serum magnesium levels. Additionally, there was a marked decrease in periodic limb movements during wakefulness and self-reported discomfort.[784]

Magnesium citrate is not actively absorbed as effectively as amino acids, which is why it may result in digestive discomfort at higher doses. To minimize these effects, it is often recommended to start at a low dose (100 to 200 mg) and gradually increase the dosage if needed. At lower doses, this form of magnesium is generally gentle and unlikely to cause urgency, loose bowel movements or gastrointestinal distress.

Magnesium Aspartate

Magnesium aspartate, a magnesium salt of aspartic acid, is used as a mineral supplement. It offers good oral bioavailability and water solubility compared to other magnesium salts like magnesium carbonate and magnesium oxide.[764, 776] Aspartate, also known as aspartic acid, is a naturally occurring amino acid that, when combined with magnesium, plays a crucial role in the production of ATP, the body's primary energy source.

A comparative study in rodents found that magnesium L-aspartate, especially when combined with vitamin B6, corrected magnesium deficiency more effectively and quicker than other tested magnesium salts.[785]

Promising clinical trials from the 1960s demonstrated that a combination of magnesium and potassium aspartates had beneficial effects on fatigue and helped reduce muscle hyper-excitability.[786] As mentioned, both magnesium and aspartic acid are essential in cellular energy production. Although this form is not commonly used or widely available, it is primarily used in situations where low energy levels and chronic fatigue syndrome are present. However, another form of magnesium, called magnesium malate, which is more readily available, also helps with these issues.

Magnesium Glycinate/Bisglycinate

Magnesium glycinate, also referred to as magnesium diglycinate or magnesium bisglycinate, is a compound formed by combining one magnesium molecule with two glycine molecules.[787] This form of magnesium offers good bioavailability without causing a laxative effect.[776] Magnesium glycinate is more effectively absorbed in the intestines compared to other forms.[788] In a study examining the dose-dependent bioavailability of various amino acid organic magnesium compounds, it was found that magnesium glycinate increased brain magnesium levels only at higher doses, while blood magnesium levels rose across all dosage levels.[763]

Glycine is an essential neurotransmitter and plays key roles in various processes such as antioxidant activity, inflammation control, metabolic health, cardiovascular diseases, diabetes, obesity, neurological functions, sleep and maintaining body homeostasis.[789] Given these benefits, magnesium glycinate has become one of the most popular supplements available today, effectively addressing a wide range of health concerns including chronic pain, anxiety, insomnia, and muscle tightness/stiffness. It's important to note however, that most of glycine's benefits occur at around the 3-to-10-gram range per day, necessitating additional glycine compared to what would be provided by magnesium glycinate. Typical doses of magnesium glycinate will only provide around 600 mg of glycine per day.

As mentioned, magnesium glycinate is known for its effectiveness in relieving muscle cramps and tightness. In a study involving eighty women, magnesium bisglycinate chelate (300 mg per day) was compared to a placebo for treating pregnancy-induced leg cramps.[790] By the fourth week, the magnesium group experienced a significantly greater reduction in cramp frequency. These findings suggest that magnesium bisglycinate may be an effective option for reducing the frequency and intensity of leg cramps during pregnancy.[790]

Magnesium has been shown to positively impact mood and mental well-being. Case histories reveal that taking 125–300 mg of magnesium (in the form of glycinate and taurinate) with each meal and before bed resulted in rapid recovery from major depression, often in less than 7 days.[418] Overall, magnesium was demonstrated to be effective in alleviating depressive symptoms.

Vitamin D is essential for overall health, playing a vital role in maintaining bone strength, supporting the immune system, and regulating cardiovascular function. Magnesium plays a crucial role in the metabolism of vitamin D. In a study by Cheung, M. M., et al. they assessed the effectiveness of a combined regimen of magnesium glycinate and vitamin D compared to vitamin D alone, focusing on their impact on increasing serum 25-hydroxyvitamin D (25OHD) levels and their effects on cardiometabolic health.[513] Their findings were that a combined magnesium glycinate and vitamin D treatment was more effective in raising serum 25OHD concentrations than vitamin D supplementation alone. They also observed a reduction in systolic blood pressure in individuals with a baseline systolic blood pressure greater than 132 mmHg within the combined magnesium glycinate and vitamin D group.[513]

In conclusion, magnesium glycinate stands out as a well-rounded form of magnesium supplementation, largely due to its combination with the amino acid glycine. Its superior absorption and the synergistic effects of glycine make it a valuable option for those seeking to optimize their magnesium intake and overall well-being. Many people find magnesium glycinate is a great option particularly for sleep.

Magnesium Taurate

Magnesium taurate is a form of magnesium combined with taurine, an amino acid that is abundant in heart muscle.[791] Magnesium taurate has good bioavailability. Taurine is a sulfur-containing amino acid abundant in the central nervous system that is known for its protective roles in the brain. It also has an anxiolytic effect by activating glycine receptors. Studies show that taurine levels in the brain increase to protect neurons, and there is a specific taurine transport system in the blood-brain barrier.

Magnesium and taurine share several similar actions that can significantly improve cardiac function, reducing high blood pressure, preventing atherosclerosis, stabilizing platelets, correcting irregular heartbeats, reducing tissue calcium buildup, improving insulin sensitivity, and potentially preventing diabetic complications.[792]

In a study involving hypertensive rats, magnesium taurate was administered orally in doses of 2 and 4 mg/kg/day.[793] The results showed that magnesium taurate significantly reduced both systolic and diastolic blood pressure and restored myocardial antioxidant levels, such as glutathione peroxidase and catalase, which were diminished by hypertension. Additionally, magnesium taurate reduced heart damage caused by hypertension, demonstrating its strong antihypertensive and cardioprotective effects, likely due to its antioxidant properties. The study concluded that magnesium taurate, with its potent antihypertensive and cardioprotective effects, could be a valuable supplement for improving cardiovascular health.[793]

In another recent study researchers evaluated the effectiveness of magnesium taurate (500 mg per day for 30 days) in reducing blood pressure in individuals with chronic hypertension.[794] Blood pressure levels significantly dropped, with systolic pressure going from 151 mmHg down to 130 mmHg and diastolic pressure going from 92.10 mmHg down to 80.30 mmHg. Additionally, the results revealed a significant decrease in cortisol levels, suggesting stress regulation.[794] These results indicate a therapeutic benefit with magnesium taurate in the management of hypertension.

In a publication by McCarty M. F., he theorized that parenteral magnesium taurate can be considered a superior alternative to magnesium sulfate in the treatment of pre-eclampsia.[795] When included as part of prenatal supplementation, McCarty believed that magnesium taurate may offer both preventive and therapeutic benefits for this syndrome. Given the hypoxia-protective properties of both magnesium and taurine, he believed that this supplementation could also help protect fetuses from temporary perinatal asphyxia, potentially reducing the risk of cerebral palsy.[795]

In conclusion, magnesium taurate is notable for its effective combination of magnesium and taurine, which work together synergistically to enhance its overall effectiveness. The complementary actions of magnesium's physiological benefits and taurine's protective properties make this combination an ideal choice for addressing various health concerns, especially cardiovascular health.

Magnesium Acetyl-Taurate

Magnesium acetyl taurate (also known as magnesium acetyl taurinate) is different than magnesium taurate in that it efficiently crosses into the brain, where it achieves high tissue concentrations.[796] It is also linked to a reduction in anxiety indicators.[796] Research indicates that brain magnesium levels rise regardless of the dose of magnesium taurate, likely due to the rapid absorption of even small amounts and the limited capacity of the taurine transport system.[763]

Recent studies are also exploring the potential of magnesium acetyl taurate in treating traumatic brain injury. In the development of traumatic brain injury, the initial damage involves mechanical injury to nerve fibers, such as laceration and stretching. This is followed by secondary damage, including ischemia, oxidative stress, and mitochondrial dysfunction. Studies have indicated that a decrease in magnesium levels contributes to these secondary damage processes. Magnesium acetyl taurate, which penetrates brain tissue effectively, shows promise as a potential treatment to prevent both structural and functional damage in traumatic brain injury.[797]

Magnesium Malate

Magnesium malate is a compound created by combining magnesium with malic acid. Malic acid (malate), is an essential component of the citric acid cycle in the mitochondria, where it plays a crucial role in energy production.[798] Magnesium malate seems to be the best magnesium supplement for increasing muscle magnesium content.[796] Magnesium malate would be the best magnesium supplement to combine with magnesium acetyl taurate, as the latter has been found to lower muscle magnesium concentrations potentially due to its ability to shunt magnesium away from skeletal muscle and into the brain.[796]

After administering a single dose of 400 mg/70 kg of magnesium to Sprague Dawley rats, researchers assessed its bioavailability by studying absorption rates, tissue penetration, and behavioral effects.[796] The results showed that magnesium malate had the highest area under the curve, indicating superior pharmacokinetic performance. Magnesium malate levels in the serum remained elevated for an extended period, demonstrating its prolonged bioavailability.[796]

As mentioned, malic acid plays a crucial role in energy production as a key precursor in ATP synthesis. This essential organic acid helps drive the citric acid cycle, which is vital for converting nutrients into energy.[799] This combination is thought to benefit individuals experiencing fibromyalgia by supporting energy production and reducing discomfort. In a study by Russell, I. J. et al., researchers tested a tablet containing malic acid (200 mg) and magnesium (50 mg) on primary fibromyalgia syndrome. The study started with a 4-week placebo-controlled trial, followed by a 6-month open-label trial with increased dosage. They found that longer treatment and higher doses significantly reduced pain and tenderness without significant risks.[800] Abraham and Flechas conducted an 8-week study involving 15 fibromyalgia patients, using a combination of magnesium (300-600 mg) and malate (1200-2400 mg) in a randomized, placebo-controlled, open-label, crossover trial. The treatment group showed improvements in their Tender Point Index scores and reported reduced muscle pain.[801]

The primary symptom of chronic fatigue syndrome is severe exhaustion, which is also a key feature of fibromyalgia.[802] Given that malic acid is crucial to the energy-producing citric acid cycle in the body, it is understandable why some people opt to supplement with it for this condition.

Aluminum interferes with energy production in cells by inhibiting glycolysis and oxidative phosphorylation, leading to decreased ATP and increased AMP levels. It also blocks phosphate absorption, causing a deficiency in mitochondrial phosphate, which is essential for ATP synthesis. However, adequate magnesium levels can prevent this toxic effect. Malic acid is a strong chelator of aluminum and has been shown to be the most effective in reducing aluminum levels in the brain.[801]

In conclusion, the role of magnesium and malic acid in enhancing energy production holds significant promise, particularly for athletes. The improved ATP production facilitated by malic acid can potentially boost endurance, while magnesium's contribution to proper muscle function further supports athletic performance.[803] Additionally, because malate (malic acid) is an amino acid, it is efficiently absorbed and generally causes minimal digestive upset.[763] Thus, the combination of magnesium and malate offers a beneficial approach for those seeking to optimize their energy levels and overall physical performance.

Magnesium Orotate

Magnesium orotate is a compound that combines magnesium with orotic acid. This form has good bioavailability and has been studied specifically for heart health.[257] Orotic acid helps transport magnesium into cells. Its antioxidant protection mainly comes from pyrimidine bases, which boost the production of enzymes that fight off free radicals.[804] The salt has low solubility in water, so it does not bind to gastric acid or cause significant laxative effects when taken orally.[805] Since orotic acid stabilizes magnesium in cells, it results in strong antiarrhythmic, vasodilating, and heart-protective effects.[806]

The involvement of orotic acid in metabolic processes explains its cardiovascular and neuroprotective effects. By increasing the resistance of heart muscle cells to a lack of oxygen, orotic acid positively impacts the course of heart attacks and reduces symptoms of heart failure. Orotic acid has been noted to have an angioprotective action and to play an important role in the energy provision of the hypertrophic myocardium, by increasing its contractility.[806] It has also been shown to enhance energy levels in damaged heart tissue by boosting the production of glycogen and ATP.[805]

Magnesium orotate, when used as an adjuvant therapy alongside optimal treatment for severe congestive heart failure, has been shown to significantly increase survival rates and improve clinical symptoms.[257] Patients were randomly assigned to receive either magnesium orotate (6000 mg for the first month, followed by 3000 mg for about 11 months) or a placebo, alongside their cardiovascular treatment. Over the course of a year, patients receiving magnesium orotate had a survival rate of 75.7% compared to 51.6% for those on placebo. Additionally, 38.5% of patients on magnesium orotate experienced symptom improvement, while 56.3% of those on placebo had a worsening of symptoms.[257]

A study evaluated the benefits of magnesium orotate with chronic ischemic heart failure after coronary artery by-pass graft surgery. They found that magnesium orotate significantly improved exercise capacity and reduced ventricular premature beats, with minimal adverse reactions.[807] In another study, patients with coronary heart disease and left ventricular dysfunction who took magnesium orotate experienced significant improvements in heart function and exercise tolerance compared to those on a placebo.[808] Finally in a double-blind randomized study involving 23 competitive triathletes, 4-week supplementation with magnesium orotate led to a significantly faster swimming time compared to a placebo. The magnesium orotate group showed improved energy metabolism, lower serum insulin and cortisol levels, reduced blood proton concentration (less acidic blood), and less muscle damage (lower creatine kinase levels) compared to the control group.[809] Some of these benefits have been proposed by DiNicolantonio and McCarty to be due to the fact that orotate is converted to beta-alanine in the body, which boosts the carnosine pool.[810]

Recent studies highlight the role of magnesium orotate in supporting the microbiome-gut-brain axis, which is linked to both mental and digestive health. In a small study, 17 patients with treatment-resistant depression were given magnesium orotate, probiotics, and a selective serotonin reuptake inhibitor (SSRI) for 8 weeks. All patients showed improved depression and anxiety scores, along with increased energy and well-being, suggesting a synergistic effect on the gut-brain axis. However, a follow-up at 16 weeks revealed a relapse when only the SSRI medication was used.[811] These results suggest that supplementing with magnesium orotate and probiotics could be beneficial for improving gut-brain health, however more research in this area is needed.

Magnesium orotate offers a unique combination of benefits, from supporting cardiovascular health to potentially enhancing mental well-being. Its role in cellular processes and the gut-brain axis highlights its importance in various therapeutic applications. Although current research is promising, further studies are needed to fully explore all its capabilities and confirm its effectiveness in other diverse health conditions.

Magnesium L-Threonate

Magnesium L-threonate is a compound created by combining magnesium with threonic acid, a water-soluble substance produced from the metabolism of vitamin C.[812] Animal studies have demonstrated that magnesium L-threonate has a unique ability to penetrate the brain and elevate magnesium levels in the cerebrospinal fluid.[493, 812] It has also been shown to help regulate synapse density, which is correlated to nerve transmission and growth.[812] Synaptic density refers to the structural health of brain synapses. Higher synaptic density leads to more efficient cognitive processing.[813] L-Threonate can boost mitochondrial function, essential proteins for synaptic plasticity, and both the number and quality of synapses.[812]

Maintaining a healthy number of synapses is crucial for brain function, as cognitive decline with age is closely linked to synapse loss. Few molecules have been found to boost synapse density, and threonate may be a key molecule in cerebrospinal fluid for sustaining high synapse density.[812] The combination of L-threonate and magnesium boosts synapse density in essential brain areas, including the prefrontal cortex and hippocampus. This enhancement supports key functions such as executive function, learning, and memory. In vivo studies showed that oral treatment with L-threonate and magnesium boosted brain threonate levels by about 50% and cerebrospinal fluid magnesium by 15%, resulting in a 67% increase in synapse density.[814] Animal studies have found that neither L-threonate or magnesium alone were effective to increase short or long-term memory ability; only their combination boosted memory.[814] Oral treatments with this combination have successfully enhanced synapse density and memory in aged rats and mice with advanced Alzheimer's disease.[815]

In 2016, a randomized, double-blind, placebo-controlled trial was conducted to evaluate magnesium L-threonate in older adults with cognitive impairment. To qualify for the study, participants needed to be between 50 and 70 years old and report issues with memory, sleep disturbances, and anxiety. Participants were randomly divided to receive either a placebo or a daily dose of 1,500-2,000 mg of magnesium L-threonate, based on their body weight, over a 12-week period.[816] Cognitive assessments were conducted prior to the start of the supplementation and were repeated at the six-week and 12-week marks for comparison. The study's results revealed that magnesium L-threonate improved magnesium levels in the body, as evidenced by increased red blood cell concentrations and urinary excretion. It also enhanced cognitive abilities, particularly in executive function and processing speed, with significant improvements by week six. The magnesium L-threonate group showed stable cognitive performance, unlike the placebo group, which had more fluctuations. Finally, and probably most interesting, is that magnesium L-threonate reversed clinical measures of brain aging, highlighting its potential role in cognitive health. The average brain age of participants taking magnesium L-threonate supplements dropped from 69.6 to 60.6 years after just six weeks, showing a nine-year reduction, which continued to 9.4 years by week 12.[816]

An open label clinical trial tested magnesium L-threonate (plus vitamin C and vitamin D) in 15 participants with mild to moderate Alzheimer's disease.[817] Participants were over 60 years of age with a Mini-Mental State Examination (MMSE) between 14 and 24 (mean baseline score of 23). Magnesium L-threonate was given at 1800 mg per day for 8 weeks. Magnesium L-threonate led to a significant improvement in MMSE score with (mean change = + 1.73 points, p = 0.035). Importantly, even 4 months after stopping magnesium L-threonate, MMSE score was still above 24 (versus baseline MMSE score of 23).[817] Thus, magnesium L-threonate was shown to improve cognition in patients with mild to moderate Alzheimer's disease.

The microbiota-gut-brain axis is gaining increasing attention in research for its potential role in various health conditions, including neurological disorders. Disturbances in the microbiota-gut-brain axis may contribute to Alzheimer's disease development.[818] In a very recent study it was found that magnesium L-threonate modulates gut microbiota, decreasing Allobaculum and increasing Bifidobacterium and Turicibacter bacteria.[819] It also repaired intestinal barrier dysfunction and influenced pathways associated with neurodegenerative diseases, suggesting potential benefits for Alzheimer's treatment. These findings suggest that magnesium L-threonate could potentially alleviate the clinical symptoms of Alzheimer's disease by influencing the microbiota-gut-brain axis in model mice, offering a promising experimental foundation for future clinical treatments of the disease.[819]

Epidemiological studies have shown a strong link between magnesium deficiency and a higher risk of developing Parkinson's disease. Researchers used a mouse model of Parkinson's to study the protective effects of magnesium L-threonate. Mice were given various doses of magnesium L-threonate for four weeks, followed by exposure to a neurotoxin that mimics Parkinson's symptoms. Magnesium L-threonate raised magnesium levels in both the blood and the cerebrospinal fluid. The mice treated with magnesium L-threonate showed less motor decline, better coordination, and reduced neuronal loss. The treatment also decreased inflammation and oxidative stress.[493]

Emerging research is beginning to explore the potential of magnesium L-threonate in treating ADHD, with initial results showing promise. A 2021 open-pilot study found that magnesium L-threonate had a significant impact on ADHD symptoms during twelve weeks of use, with nearly half (47%) of participants showing a 25% reduction in symptoms and reporting noticeable improvement. [820]

While research into magnesium L-threonate has primarily focused on its effects on learning, cognitive decline, and memory, most of these studies have been conducted in animal models. Only a limited number of studies have involved human subjects, highlighting the need for further investigation to fully understand its potential benefits. Promisingly, emerging research is expanding to explore the impact of magnesium L-threonate on a broader range of conditions, including mood disorders, anxiety, and traumatic brain injuries. As these new studies progress, they may reveal additional therapeutic applications and provide deeper insights into how magnesium L-threonate can enhance overall mental health and well-being.

Magnesium Sulfate

Magnesium sulfate, commonly known as Epsom salts, is widely recognized for its use in various therapeutic applications, including in bath soaks for muscle relaxation. However, most of the research surrounding magnesium sulfate focuses on its intravenous administration, which is used primarily in clinical settings for conditions such as preeclampsia[821] and certain cardiac arrhythmias.[822] This method of administration provides a rapid and controlled delivery of magnesium, but it is not readily accessible for everyday use by the general public. Consequently, while the clinical benefits of intravenous magnesium sulfate are well-documented, there is less research available on the effectiveness of topical forms of magnesium sulfate, such as Epsom salts, for broader health applications.

One study evaluated the efficacy of Epsom salt with hot water for pain relief and functional improvement in arthritis patients at a hospital. Over a 10-day period, the intervention was administered twice daily. The data was collected using the Numerical Pain Rating Scale (NPRS) and a modified Western Ontario and McMaster Universities Osteoarthritis Index (WOMAC).[823] The WOMAC index helps clinicians and researchers assess the severity of arthritis symptoms and monitor changes in response to treatment. The study found that Epsom salt with hot water significantly reduced pain and improved function, suggesting it could be a valuable non-pharmacological option to help alleviate arthritis-related discomfort.[823]

Although research on Epsom salts is limited, they are generally considered safe and may offer benefits for joint and muscle relief, as well as overall relaxation. This soothing effect not only aids in physical comfort but can also support mental well-being, making Epsom salts a simple yet potentially valuable addition to self-care routines.

Final Conclusions

As we conclude this book, it is evident that magnesium is an essential mineral crucial to our health and well-being. We have examined its essential roles in various bodily functions, from supporting muscle and nerve activity to regulating blood pressure and maintaining bone health. Each form of magnesium offers distinct benefits, highlighting the mineral's broad impact on our overall health.

Despite its importance, magnesium deficiency is alarmingly common and represents a significant public health crisis. Many individuals are not meeting their daily magnesium needs. This can lead to a range of health problems, everything from fatigue and muscle cramps to more serious conditions like cardiovascular disease and diabetes. Addressing this widespread deficiency is crucial for improving public health and ensuring that everyone can benefit from this essential mineral.

How To Restore Magnesium Levels: 4 Step Magnesium Fix Plan

1. Identify the factors contributing to magnesium depletion. (see Chapter 1)

2. Incorporate a magnesium-rich diet into your daily routine. (see Chapter 7)

3. Determine if you are still magnesium deficient (being on the low end on serum magnesium levels, magnesium deficiency symptoms and/or low magnesium in the urine - See Chapter 1).

4. Consider the option of magnesium supplementation.

Our primary goal in writing this book was to inform and raise awareness about the expanding body of research highlighting the crucial role magnesium plays in maintaining overall health. Magnesium is often overlooked and commonly referred to as the "missing mineral," yet its impact on our health is truly profound. Our aim is to inspire action toward addressing the widespread deficiency and ensuring magnesium becomes a true partner in supporting better health outcomes. Magnesium is not just necessary—it is *essential* for the health of our entire body.

References

1. DiNicolantonio, J.J., J.H. O'Keefe, and W. Wilson, *Subclinical magnesium deficiency: a principal driver of cardiovascular disease and a public health crisis.* Open Heart, 2018. **5**(1): p. e000668.

2. Souza, A.C.R., et al., *The Integral Role of Magnesium in Muscle Integrity and Aging: A Comprehensive Review.* Nutrients, 2023. **15**(24).

3. *Sakula A. Doctor Nehemiah Grew (1641-1712) and the Epsom salts. Clio Med. 1984;19(1-2):1-21. PMID: 6085985.*

4. *National Center for Biotechnology Information (2024). PubChem Element Summary for AtomicNumber 12, Magnesium. Retrieved March 17, 2024 from https://pubchem.ncbi.nlm.nih.gov/element/Magnesium.*

5. *LeroyJ. Necessite du magnesium pour la croissance de la souris. CR Soc Biol 94: 431, 1926.*

6. Seelig, M.S., *THE REQUIREMENT OF MAGNESIUM BY THE NORMAL ADULT. SUMMARY AND ANALYSIS OF PUBLISHED DATA.* Am J Clin Nutr, 1964. **14**: p. 242-90.

7. DiNicolantonio, J.J., M.F. McCarty, and J.H. O'Keefe, *Decreased magnesium status may mediate the increased cardiovascular risk associated with calcium supplementation.* Open Heart, 2017. **4**(1): p. e000617.

8. de Baaij, J.H., J.G. Hoenderop, and R.J. Bindels, *Magnesium in man: implications for health and disease.* Physiol Rev, 2015. **95**(1): p. 1-46.

9. Vormann, J., *Magnesium: nutrition and metabolism.* Mol Aspects Med, 2003. **24**(1-3): p. 27-37.

10. Wacker, W.E. and A.F. Parisi, *Magnesium metabolism.* N Engl J Med, 1968. **278**(12): p. 658-63.

11. Abbott, L.G. and R.K. Rude, *Clinical manifestations of magnesium deficiency.* Miner Electrolyte Metab, 1993. **19**(4-5): p. 314-22.

12. Rude, R.K. and H.E. Gruber, *Magnesium deficiency and osteoporosis: animal and human observations.* J Nutr Biochem, 2004. **15**(12): p. 710-6.

13. Smith, R.H., *Calcium and magnesium metabolism in calves. 4. Bone composition in magnesium deficiency and the control of plasma magnesium.* Biochem J, 1959. **71**(4): p. 609-14.

14. Yasui, M., Y. Yase, and K. Ota, *[Evaluation of magnesium, calcium and aluminum deposition in bone in situ].* No To Shinkei, 1991. **43**(6): p. 577-82.

15. Ubom, G.A., *The goitre-soil-water-diet relationship: case study in Plateau State, Nigeria.* Sci Total Environ, 1991. **107**: p. 1-11.

16. Louzada, M.L., et al., *Impact of ultra-processed foods on micronutrient content in the Brazilian diet.* Rev Saude Publica, 2015. **49**: p. 45.

17. Marier, J.R., *Magnesium content of the food supply in the modern-day world.* Magnesium, 1986. **5**(1): p. 1-8.

18. Hermes Sales, C., et al., *There is chronic latent magnesium deficiency in apparently healthy university students.* Nutr Hosp, 2014. **30**(1): p. 200-4.

19. Elin, R.J., *Re-evaluation of the concept of chronic, latent, magnesium deficiency.* Magnes Res, 2011. **24**(4): p. 225-7.

20. Durlach, J., *Recommended dietary amounts of magnesium: Mg RDA*. Magnes Res, 1989. **2**(3): p. 195-203.

21. Gillis, L. and A. Gillis, *Nutrient inadequacy in obese and non-obese youth*. Can J Diet Pract Res, 2005. **66**(4): p. 237-42.

22. Wang, J.L., et al., *Magnesium status and association with diabetes in the Taiwanese elderly*. Asia Pac J Clin Nutr, 2005. **14**(3): p. 263-9.

23. Itokawa, Y., *[Magnesium intake and cardiovascular disease]*. Clin Calcium, 2005. **15**(2): p. 154-9.

24. Rosanoff, A., C.M. Weaver, and R.K. Rude, *Suboptimal magnesium status in the United States: are the health consequences underestimated?* Nutr Rev, 2012. **70**(3): p. 153-64.

25. Costello, R.B., et al., *Perspective: The Case for an Evidence-Based Reference Interval for Serum Magnesium: The Time Has Come*. Advances in Nutrition, 2016. **7**: p. 977-993.

26. Lakshmanan, F.L., et al., *Magnesium intakes, balances, and blood levels of adults consuming self-selected diets*. Am J Clin Nutr, 1984. **40**(6 Suppl): p. 1380-9.

27. Tipton, I.H., P.L. Stewart, and J. Dickson, *Patterns of elemental excretion in long term balance studies*. Health Phys, 1969. **16**(4): p. 455-62.

28. Hunt, C.D. and L.K. Johnson, *Magnesium requirements: new estimations for men and women by cross-sectional statistical analyses of metabolic magnesium balance data*. Am J Clin Nutr, 2006. **84**(4): p. 843-52.

29. Vormann, J. and M. Anke, *Dietary magnesium: supply, requirements and recommendations--results from duplicate and balance studies in man*. J. Clin. Basic Cardiol, 2002. **5**(49-53).

30. Davydenko, N.V. and I.G. Vasilenko, *[Magnesium level in food rations and the prevalence of ischemic heart disease among the population]*. Gig Sanit, 1991(5): p. 44-6.

31. Durlach, J., *New data on the importance of gestational Mg deficiency*. J Am Coll Nutr, 2004. **23**(6): p. 694s-700s.

32. Carriere, I., et al., *Nutrient intake in an elderly population in southern France (POLANUT): deficiency in some vitamins, minerals and omega-3 PUFA*. Int J Vitam Nutr Res, 2007. **77**(1): p. 57-65.

33. Henzel, J.H., M.S. DeWeese, and G. Ridenhour, *Significance of magnesium and zinc metabolism in the surgical patient. I. Magnesium*. Arch Surg, 1967. **95**(6): p. 974-90.

34. ter Borg, S., et al., *Micronutrient intakes and potential inadequacies of community-dwelling older adults: a systematic review*. Br J Nutr, 2015. **113**(8): p. 1195-206.

35. Cohen, L. and R. Kitzes, *Infrared spectroscopy and magnesium content of bone mineral in osteoporotic women*. Isr J Med Sci, 1981. **17**(12): p. 1123-5.

36. Lima Mde, L., et al., *[Magnesium deficiency and insulin resistance in patients with type 2 diabetes mellitus]*. Arq Bras Endocrinol Metabol, 2005. **49**(6): p. 959-63.

37. Touitou, Y., et al., *Prevalence of magnesium and potassium deficiencies in the elderly*. Clin Chem, 1987. **33**(4): p. 518-23.

38. Caddell, J.L., *Magnesium deficiency in man*. Del Med J, 1968. **40**(5): p. 133-8.

39. Dorup, I. and K. Skajaa, *[Magnesium and long-term diuretic therapy]*. Ugeskr Laeger, 1989. **151**(12): p. 759-63.

40. Malon, A., et al., *Ionized magnesium in erythrocytes--the best magnesium parameter to observe hypo- or hypermagnesemia*. Clin Chim Acta, 2004. **349**(1-2): p. 67-73.

41. Ryzen, E., *Magnesium homeostasis in critically ill patients.* Magnesium, 1989. **8**(3-4): p. 201-12.

42. Rubeiz, G.J., et al., *Association of hypomagnesemia and mortality in acutely ill medical patients.* Crit Care Med, 1993. **21**(2): p. 203-9.

43. Olerich, M.A. and R.K. Rude, *Should we supplement magnesium in critically ill patients?* New Horiz, 1994. **2**(2): p. 186-92.

44. Gullestad, L., et al., *Magnesium deficiency diagnosed by an intravenous loading test.* Scand J Clin Lab Invest, 1992. **52**(4): p. 245-53.

45. Seelig, C.B., *Magnesium deficiency in two hypertensive patient groups.* South Med J, 1990. **83**(7): p. 739-42.

46. Malini, P.L., et al., *Angiotensin converting enzyme inhibitors, thiazide diuretics and magnesium balance. A preliminary study.* Magnes Res, 1990. **3**(3): p. 193-6.

47. Cohen, L. and A. Laor, *Correlation between bone magnesium concentration and magnesium retention in the intravenous magnesium load test.* Magnes Res, 1990. **3**(4): p. 271-4.

48. Dolev, E., et al., *Longitudinal study of magnesium status of Israeli military recruits.* Magnes Trace Elem, 1991. **10**(5-6): p. 420-6.

49. Buchman, A.L., et al., *The effect of a marathon run on plasma and urine mineral and metal concentrations.* J Am Coll Nutr, 1998. **17**(2): p. 124-7.

50. Spatling, L., et al., *[Diagnosing magnesium deficiency. Current recommendations of the Society for Magnesium Research].* Fortschr Med Orig, 2000. **118 Suppl 2**: p. 49-53.

51. Whang, R., *Routine serum magnesium determination--a continuing unrecognized need.* Magnesium, 1987. **6**(1): p. 1-4.

52. Liebscher, D.H. and D.E. Liebscher, *About the misdiagnosis of magnesium deficiency.* J Am Coll Nutr, 2004. **23**(6): p. 730s-1s.

53. Slatopolsky, E., et al., *The hypocalcemia of magnesium depletion.* Adv Exp Med Biol, 1978. **103**: p. 263-71.

54. Nielsen, F.H., et al., *Moderate magnesium deprivation results in calcium retention and altered potassium and phosphorus excretion by postmenopausal women.* Magnes Res, 2007. **20**(1): p. 19-31.

55. *Vormann, J., Anke, M., 2002. Dietary magnesium: supply, requirements and recommendations—results from duplicate and balance studies in man. J. Clin. Basic Cardiol. 5, 49–53.*

56. Nielsen, F.H. and D.B. Milne, *Some magnesium status indicators and oxidative metabolism responses to low-dietary magnesium are affected by dietary copper in postmenopausal women.* Nutrition, 2003. **19**(7-8): p. 617-26.

57. Spencer, H., et al., *Effect of magnesium on the intestinal absorption of calcium in man.* J Am Coll Nutr, 1994. **13**(5): p. 485-92.

58. *Professional, C. C. medical. (n.d.). Hypomagnesemia: What it is, causes, symptoms & treatment. Cleveland Clinic. https://my.clevelandclinic.org/health/diseases/23264-hypomagnesemia.*

59. *Carabotti, M., Annibale, B., & Lahner, E. (2021). Common pitfalls in the management of patients with micronutrient deficiency: Keep in mind the stomach. Nutrients, 13(1), 208.*

60. Kieboom, B.C., et al., *Proton pump inhibitors and hypomagnesemia in the general population: a population-based cohort study.* Am J Kidney Dis, 2015. **66**(5): p. 775-82.

61. *Bruley des Varannes, S. Proton pump inhibitors in gastroesophageal reflux disease. Frontiers of Gastrointestinal Research. 2013. 34–46.*

62. DiNicolantonio, J.J. and J. O'Keefe, *Low-grade metabolic acidosis as a driver of chronic disease: a 21st century public health crisis.* Open Heart, 2021. **8**(2).

63. *Magnesium deficiency.* Br Med J, 1967. **2**(5546): p. 195.

64. Uğurlu, V., et al., *Cellular Trace Element Changes in Type 1 Diabetes Patients.* J Clin Res Pediatr Endocrinol, 2016. **8**(2): p. 180-6.

65. Schnack, C., et al., *Hypomagnesaemia in type 2 (non-insulin-dependent) diabetes mellitus is not corrected by improvement of long-term metabolic control.* Diabetologia, 1992. **35**(1): p. 77-9.

66. Kraut, J.A. and N.E. Madias, *Metabolic acidosis: pathophysiology, diagnosis and management.* Nat Rev Nephrol, 2010. **6**(5): p. 274-85.

67. Rylander, R., et al., *Acid-base status affects renal magnesium losses in healthy, elderly persons.* J Nutr, 2006. **136**(9): p. 2374-7.

68. *McKay, C. P. (Disorders of magnesium metabolism. Fluid and Electrolytes in Pediatrics. 2009. 149–171. https://doi.org/10.1007/978-1-60327-225-4_5.*

69. Pickering, G., et al., *Magnesium Status and Stress: The Vicious Circle Concept Revisited.* Nutrients, 2020. **12**(12).

70. Seelig, M.S., *Consequences of magnesium deficiency on the enhancement of stress reactions; preventive and therapeutic implications (a review).* J Am Coll Nutr, 1994. **13**(5): p. 429-46.

71. Gröber, U., *Magnesium and Drugs.* Int J Mol Sci, 2019. **20**(9).

72. Hollifield, J.W., *Magnesium depletion, diuretics, and arrhythmias.* Am J Med, 1987. **82**(3a): p. 30-7.

73. Kynast-Gales, S.A. and L.K. Massey, *Effect of caffeine on circadian excretion of urinary calcium and magnesium.* J Am Coll Nutr, 1994. **13**(5): p. 467-72.

74. Bergman, E.A., et al., *Effects of dietary caffeine on renal handling of minerals in adult women.* Life Sci, 1990. **47**(6): p. 557-64.

75. Cazzola, R., et al., *Going to the roots of reduced magnesium dietary intake: A tradeoff between climate changes and sources.* Heliyon, 2020. **6**(11): p. e05390.

76. Guoa, W., et al., *Magnesium deficiency in plants: An urgent problem.* The Crop Journal, 2016. **4**(2): p. 83-91.

77. Booth, C.C., et al., *Incidence of hypomagnesaemia in intestinal malabsorption.* Br Med J, 1963. **2**(5350): p. 141-4.

78. Rude, R.K., F.R. Singer, and H.E. Gruber, *Skeletal and hormonal effects of magnesium deficiency.* J Am Coll Nutr, 2009. **28**(2): p. 131-41.

79. Richardson, J.A. and L.G. Welt, *THE HYPOMAGNESEMIA OF VITAMIN D ADMINISTRATION.* Proc Soc Exp Biol Med, 1965. **118**: p. 512-4.

80. La, S.A., et al., *Low Magnesium Levels in Adults with Metabolic Syndrome: a Meta-Analysis.* Biol Trace Elem Res, 2016. **170**(1): p. 33-42.

81. O'Hearn, M., et al., *Trends and Disparities in Cardiometabolic Health Among U.S. Adults, 1999-2018.* J Am Coll Cardiol, 2022. **80**(2): p. 138-151.

82. DiNicolantonio, J.J. and O.K. JH, *Added sugars drive coronary heart disease via insulin resistance and hyperinsulinaemia: a new paradigm.* Open Heart, 2017. **4**(2): p. e000729.

83. DiNicolantonio, J.J., J.H. O'Keefe, and S.C. Lucan, *Added Fructose: A Principal Driver of Type 2 Diabetes Mellitus and Its Consequences.* Mayo Clin Proc, 2015. **90**(3): p. 372-381.

84. Hwang, D.L., C.F. Yen, and J.L. Nadler, *Insulin increases intracellular magnesium transport in human platelets.* J Clin Endocrinol Metab, 1993. **76**(3): p. 549-53.

85. Günther, T., *The biochemical function of Mg^2+ in insulin secretion, insulin signal transduction and insulin resistance.* Magnes Res, 2010. **23**(1): p. 5-18.

86. Hosseini Dastgerdi, A., M. Ghanbari Rad, and N. Soltani, *The Therapeutic Effects of Magnesium in Insulin Secretion and Insulin Resistance.* Adv Biomed Res, 2022. **11**: p. 54.

87. Djurhuus, M.S., et al., *Insulin increases renal magnesium excretion: a possible cause of magnesium depletion in hyperinsulinaemic states.* Diabet Med, 1995. **12**(8): p. 664-9.

88. Sakhaee, K. *The effects of diuretics on magnesium metabolism. Diuretic Agents. 1997. 611–619.*

89. Lukaski, H.C., *Magnesium, zinc, and chromium nutrition and athletic performance.* Can J Appl Physiol, 2001. **26 Suppl**: p. S13-22.

90. Nishimuta, M., et al., *Dietary Salt (Sodium Chloride) Requirement and Adverse Effects of Salt Restriction in Humans.* J Nutr Sci Vitaminol (Tokyo), 2018. **64**(2): p. 83-89.

91. Vizinova, H., et al., *[The oral magnesium loading test for detecting possible magnesium deficiency].* Cas Lek Cesk, 1993. **132**(19): p. 587-9.

92. Seelig, M.S., *THE REQUIREMENT OF MAGNESIUM BY THE NORMAL ADULT. SUMMARY AND ANALYSIS OF PUBLISHED DATA.* Am J Clin Nutr, 1964. **14**(6): p. 242-90.

93. Lalor, B.C., et al., *Bone and mineral metabolism and chronic alcohol abuse.* Q J Med, 1986. **59**(229): p. 497-511.

94. Delva, P., et al., *Intralymphocyte free magnesium in patients with primary aldosteronism: aldosterone and lymphocyte magnesium homeostasis.* Hypertension, 2000. **35**(1 Pt 1): p. 113-7.

95. Mountokalakis, T.D., *Effects of aging, chronic disease, and multiple supplements on magnesium requirements.* Magnesium, 1987. **6**(1): p. 5-11.

96. Fernandez-Fernandez, F.J., et al., *Intermittent use of pantoprazole and famotidine in severe hypomagnesaemia due to omeprazole.* Neth J Med, 2010. **68**(10): p. 329-30.

97. Lipner, A., *Symptomatic magnesium deficiency after small-intestinal bypass for obesity.* Br Med J, 1977. **1**(6054): p. 148.

98. Johnson, S., *The multifaceted and widespread pathology of magnesium deficiency.* Med Hypotheses, 2001. **56**(2): p. 163-70.

99. Lum, G., *Hypomagnesemia in acute and chronic care patient populations.* Am J Clin Pathol, 1992. **97**(6): p. 827-30.

100. Rujner, J., et al., *[Magnesium status in children and adolescents with celiac disease].* Wiad Lek, 2001. **54**(5-6): p. 277-85.

101. Normen, L., et al., *Small bowel absorption of magnesium and calcium sulphate from a natural mineral water in subjects with ileostomy.* Eur J Nutr, 2006. **45**(2): p. 105-12.

102. Takase, B., et al., *Effect of chronic stress and sleep deprivation on both flow-mediated dilation in the brachial artery and the intracellular magnesium level in humans.* Clin Cardiol, 2004. **27**(4): p. 223-7.

103. Schilsky, R.L. and T. Anderson, *Hypomagnesemia and renal magnesium wasting in patients receiving cisplatin.* Ann Intern Med, 1979. **90**(6): p. 929-31.

104. Lam, M. and D.J. Adelstein, *Hypomagnesemia and renal magnesium wasting in patients treated with cisplatin.* Am J Kidney Dis, 1986. **8**(3): p. 164-9.

105. Bianchetti, M.G., et al., *Chronic renal magnesium loss, hypocalciuria and mild hypokalaemic metabolic alkalosis after cisplatin.* Pediatr Nephrol, 1990. **4**(3): p. 219-22.

106. Evans, T.R., et al., *A randomised study to determine whether routine intravenous magnesium supplements are necessary in patients receiving cisplatin chemotherapy with continuous infusion 5-fluorouracil.* Eur J Cancer, 1995. **31a**(2): p. 174-8.

107. Mashhadi, M.A., Z. Heidari, and Z. Zakeri, *Mild hypomagnesemia as the most common Cisplatin nephropathy in Iran.* Iran J Kidney Dis, 2013. **7**(1): p. 23-7.

108. Main, A.N., et al., *Mg deficiency in chronic inflammatory bowel disease and requirements during intravenous nutrition.* JPEN J Parenter Enteral Nutr, 1981. **5**(1): p. 15-9.

109. Barton, C.H., et al., *Hypomagnesemia and renal magnesium wasting in renal transplant recipients receiving cyclosporine.* Am J Med, 1987. **83**(4): p. 693-9.

110. Nozue, T., et al., *Pathogenesis of cyclosporine-induced hypomagnesemia.* J Pediatr, 1992. **120**(4 Pt 1): p. 638-40.

111. Millane, T., et al., *Mitochondrial calcium deposition in association with cyclosporine therapy and myocardial magnesium depletion: a serial histologic study in heart transplant recipients.* J Heart Lung Transplant, 1994. **13**(3): p. 473-80.

112. Rob, P.M., et al., *Myocardial magnesium depletion during cyclosporine treatment, associated with reciprocal calcium overload, can be prevented by plentiful dietary magnesium supply.* Clin Investig, 1994. **72**(2): p. 137.

113. Roffi, M., et al., *Hypermagnesiuria in children with newly diagnosed insulin-dependent diabetes mellitus.* Am J Nephrol, 1994. **14**(3): p. 201-6.

114. Revusova, V., et al., *[A decrease in magnesium in the serum and blood lymphocytes after intravenous infusion of glucose].* Cas Lek Cesk, 1991. **130**(16-17): p. 513-5.

115. Martin, B.J., J.K. McAlpine, and B.L. Devine, *Hypomagnesaemia in elderly digitalised patients.* Scott Med J, 1988. **33**(3): p. 273-4.

116. *Diuretics in the elderly.* Br Med J, 1978. **1**(6125): p. 1484.

117. Zumkley, H., et al., *Effects of drugs on magnesium requirements.* Magnesium, 1987. **6**(1): p. 12-7.

118. Cocco, G., et al., *Magnesium depletion in patients on long-term chlorthalidone therapy for essential hypertension.* Eur J Clin Pharmacol, 1987. **32**(4): p. 335-8.

119. Joo Suk, O., *Paradoxical hypomagnesemia caused by excessive ingestion of magnesium hydroxide.* Am J Emerg Med, 2008. **26**(7): p. 837.e1-2.

120. Galland, L., *Magnesium, stress and neuropsychiatric disorders.* Magnes Trace Elem, 1991. **10**(2-4): p. 287-301.

121. Kamble, T.K. and D.S. Ookalkar, *Lactational hypomagnesaemia.* Lancet, 1989. **2**(8655): p. 155-6.

122. Drenick, E.J., I.F. Hunt, and M.E. Swendseid, *Magnesium depletion during prolonged fasting of obese males.* J Clin Endocrinol Metab, 1969. **29**(10): p. 1341-8.

123. Martin, K.J., E.A. Gonzalez, and E. Slatopolsky, *Clinical consequences and management of hypomagnesemia.* J Am Soc Nephrol, 2009. **20**(11): p. 2291-5.

124. Nanji, A.A. and J.F. Denegri, *Hypomagnesemia associated with gentamicin therapy.* Drug Intell Clin Pharm, 1984. **18**(7-8): p. 596-8.

125. Zaloga, G.P., et al., *Hypomagnesemia is a common complication of aminoglycoside therapy.* Surg Gynecol Obstet, 1984. **158**(6): p. 561-5.

126. Gluszek, J., et al., *[Magnesium deficiency in tubular acidosis].* Wiad Lek, 1980. **33**(5): p. 401-4.

127. Bianchetti, M.G., O.H. Oetliker, and J. Lutschg, *Magnesium deficiency in primary distal tubular acidosis.* J Pediatr, 1993. **122**(5 Pt 1): p. 833.

128. Brannan, P.G., et al., *Magnesium absorption in the human small intestine. Results in normal subjects, patients with chronic renal disease, and patients with absorptive hypercalciuria.* J Clin Invest, 1976. **57**(6): p. 1412-8.

129. Ohtsuka, S. and I. Yamaguchi, *[Magnesium in congestive heart failure].* Clin Calcium, 2005. **15**(2): p. 181-6.

130. Vitale, C., et al., *[Mineral balance during hemodialysis and hemodiafiltration].* Minerva Urol Nefrol, 1990. **42**(3): p. 173-6.

131. Kodama, N., M. Nishimuta, and K. Suzuki, *Negative balance of calcium and magnesium under relatively low sodium intake in humans.* J Nutr Sci Vitaminol (Tokyo), 2003. **49**(3): p. 201-9.

132. Sjogren, A., C.H. Floren, and A. Nilsson, *Evaluation of magnesium status in Crohn's disease as assessed by intracellular analysis and intravenous magnesium infusion.* Scand J Gastroenterol, 1988. **23**(5): p. 555-61.

133. Oralewska, B., et al., *Disorders of magnesium homeostasis in the course of liver disease in children.* Magnes Res, 1996. **9**(2): p. 125-8.

134. Rylander, R., T. Tallheden, and J. Vormann, *Acid-base conditions regulate calcium and magnesium homeostasis.* Magnes Res, 2009. **22**(4): p. 262-5.

135. Ryzen, E. and R.K. Rude, *Low intracellular magnesium in patients with acute pancreatitis and hypocalcemia.* West J Med, 1990. **152**(2): p. 145-8.

136. Papazachariou, I.M., et al., *Magnesium deficiency in patients with chronic pancreatitis identified by an intravenous loading test.* Clin Chim Acta, 2000. **302**(1-2): p. 145-54.

137. Liamis, G., C. Gianoutsos, and M. Elisaf, *Acute pancreatitis-induced hypomagnesemia.* Pancreatology, 2001. **1**(1): p. 74-6.

138. Bhardwaj, P., et al., *Micronutrient antioxidant intake in patients with chronic pancreatitis.* Trop Gastroenterol, 2004. **25**(2): p. 69-72.

139. Markell, M.S., et al., *Deficiency of serum ionized magnesium in patients receiving hemodialysis or peritoneal dialysis.* Asaio j, 1993. **39**(3): p. M801-4.

140. Shabajee, N., et al., *Omeprazole and refractory hypomagnesaemia.* Bmj, 2008. **337**: p. a425.

141. Mackay, J.D. and P.T. Bladon, *Hypomagnesaemia due to proton-pump inhibitor therapy: a clinical case series.* Qjm, 2010. **103**(6): p. 387-95.

142. Stendig-Lindberg, G., et al., *Changes in serum magnesium concentration after strenuous exercise.* J Am Coll Nutr, 1987. **6**(1): p. 35-40.

143. Turnlund, J.R., et al., *Vitamin B-6 depletion followed by repletion with animal- or plant-source diets and calcium and magnesium metabolism in young women.* Am J Clin Nutr, 1992. **56**(5): p. 905-10.

144. Spasov, A.A., et al., *Features of central neurotransmission in animals in conditions of dietary magnesium deficiency and after its correction.* Neurosci Behav Physiol, 2009. **39**(7): p. 645-53.

145. Hanna, S., *Influence of large doses of vitamin D on magnesium metabolism in rats.* Metabolism, 1961. **10**: p. 735-43.

146. *https://en.wikipedia.org/wiki/Trousseau_sign_of_latent_tetany.*

147. Shils, M.E., *Experimental human magnesium depletion.* Medicine (Baltimore), 1969. **48**(1): p. 61-85.

148. Grobin, W., *A New Syndrome, Magnesium-Deficiency Tetany.* Can Med Assoc J, 1960. **82**(20): p. 1034-5.

149. Gerst, P.H., M.R. Porter, and R.A. Fishman, *SYMPTOMATIC MAGNESIUM DEFICIENCY IN SURGICAL PATIENTS.* Ann Surg, 1964. **159**: p. 402-6.

150. *https://www.google.com/#q=fasciculations.*

151. Alloui, A., et al., *Does Mg2+ deficiency induce a long-term sensitization of the central nociceptive pathways?* Eur J Pharmacol, 2003. **469**(1-3): p. 65-9.

152. Durlach, J., et al., *Headache due to photosensitive magnesium depletion.* Magnes Res, 2005. **18**(2): p. 109-22.

153. Cevette, M.J., et al., *Phase 2 study examining magnesium-dependent tinnitus.* Int Tinnitus J, 2011. **16**(2): p. 168-73.

154. Agarwal, R., et al., *Mechanisms of cataractogenesis in the presence of magnesium deficiency.* Magnes Res, 2013. **26**(1): p. 2-8.

155. McCoy, J.H. and M.A. Kenney, *Depressed immune response in the magnesium-deficient rat.* J Nutr, 1975. **105**(6): p. 791-7.

156. Siwek, M., et al., *[The role of copper and magnesium in the pathogenesis and treatment of affective disorders].* Psychiatr Pol, 2005. **39**(5): p. 911-20.

157. Cevette, M.J., J. Vormann, and K. Franz, *Magnesium and hearing.* J Am Acad Audiol, 2003. **14**(4): p. 202-12.

158. Kitlinski, M., et al., *Is magnesium deficit in lymphocytes a part of the mitral valve prolapse syndrome?* Magnes Res, 2004. **17**(1): p. 39-45.

159. Rude, R.K., S.B. Oldham, and F.R. Singer, *Functional hypoparathyroidism and parathyroid hormone end-organ resistance in human magnesium deficiency.* Clin Endocrinol (Oxf), 1976. **5**(3): p. 209-24.

160. Jooste, P.L., et al., *Epileptic-type convulsions and magnesium deficiency.* Aviat Space Environ Med, 1979. **50**(7): p. 734-5.

161. Canelas, H.M., L.M. De Assis, and F.B. De Jorge, *DISORDERS OF MAGNESIUM METABOLISM IN EPILEPSY.* J Neurol Neurosurg Psychiatry, 1965. **28**: p. 378-81.

162. Vitale, J.J., et al., *Magnesium deficiency in the Cebus monkey.* Circ Res, 1963. **12**: p. 642-50.

163. Spisak, V., *[Magnesium loading test in cardiovascular diseases].* Vnitr Lek, 1992. **38**(4): p. 337-44.

164. Gullestad, L., et al., *The magnesium loading test: reference values in healthy subjects.* Scand J Clin Lab Invest, 1994. **54**(1): p. 23-31.

165. Gullestad, L., et al., *Magnesium status in healthy free-living elderly Norwegians.* J Am Coll Nutr, 1994. **13**(1): p. 45-50.

166. Sjögren, A., C.H. Floren, and A. Nilsson, *Measurements of magnesium in mononuclear cells.* Sci Total Environ, 1985. **42**(1-2): p. 77-82.

167. Hosseini, J.M., J.E. Niemela, and R.J. Elin, *Mononuclear blood cell magnesium in older subjects: evaluation of its use in clinical practice.* Ann Clin Biochem, 1995. **32 (Pt 4)**: p. 435.

168. Lim, P., et al., *Values for tissue magnesium as a guide in detecting magnesium deficiency.* J Clin Pathol, 1969. **22**(4): p. 417-21.

169. Kozielec, T., et al., *The influence of magnesium supplementation on magnesium and calcium concentrations in hair of children with magnesium shortage.* Magnes Res, 2001. **14**(1-2): p. 33-8.

170. Solarska, K., M. Stepniewski, and J. Pach, *Concentration of magnesium in hair of inhabitants of down-town Krakow, the protective zone of Steel-Mill "Huta im. Sendzimira" and Tokarnia village.* Przegl Lek, 1995. **52**(5): p. 263-6.

171. Vormann, J. and M. Anke, *Dietary magnesium: supply, requirements and recommendations—results from duplicate and balance studies in man.* J. Clin. Basic Cardiol, 2002. **5**: p. 49-53.

172. Durlach, J., et al., *Importance of the ratio between ionized and total Mg in serum or plasma: new data on the regulation of Mg status and practical importance of total Mg concentration in the investigation of Mg imbalance.* Magnes Res, 2002. **15**(3-4): p. 203-5.

173. Rude, R.K., A. Stephen, and J. Nadler, *Determination of red blood cell intracellular free magnesium by nuclear magnetic resonance as an assessment of magnesium depletion.* Magnes Trace Elem, 1991. **10**(2-4): p. 117-21.

174. Markell, M.S., et al., *Ionized and total magnesium levels in cyclosporin-treated renal transplant recipients: relationship with cholesterol and cyclosporin levels.* Clin Sci (Lond), 1993. **85**(3): p. 315-8.

175. Thomas, J., et al., *Free and total magnesium in lymphocytes of migraine patients - effect of magnesium-rich mineral water intake.* Clin Chim Acta, 2000. **295**(1-2): p. 63-75.

176. Elisaf, M., et al., *Fractional excretion of magnesium in normal subjects and in patients with hypomagnesemia.* Magnes Res, 1997. **10**(4): p. 315-20.

177. Assadi, F., *Hypomagnesemia: an evidence-based approach to clinical cases.* Iran J Kidney Dis, 2010. **4**(1): p. 13-9.

178. Nadler, J.L., et al., *Intracellular free magnesium deficiency plays a key role in increased platelet reactivity in type II diabetes mellitus.* Diabetes Care, 1992. **15**(7): p. 835-41.

179. Ismail, A.A.A., Y. Ismail, and A.A. Ismail, *Chronic magnesium deficiency and human disease; time for reappraisal?* Qjm, 2018. **111**(11): p. 759-763.

180. Morris, J.N., M.D. Crawford, and J.A. Heady, *Hardness of local water-supplies and mortality from cardiovascular disease in the County Boroughs of England and Wales.* Lancet, 1961. **1**(7182): p. 860-2.

181. Crawford, M.D., M.J. Gardner, and J.N. Morris, *Mortality and hardness of local water-supplies.* Lancet, 1968. **1**(7547): p. 827-31.

182. Masironi, R. and A.G. Shaper, *Epidemiological studies of health effects of water from different sources.* Annu Rev Nutr, 1981. **1**: p. 375-400.

183. Greathouse, D.G. and R.H. Osborne, *Preliminary report on nationwide study of drinking water and cardiovascular diseases.* J Environ Pathol Toxicol, 1980. **4**(2-3): p. 65-76.

184. *Define mono-valent, divalent and trivalent elements with example. Unacademy. (2022, June 21). https://unacademy.com/content/question-answer/chemistry/define-mono-valent-divalent-and-trivalent-elements-with-example/#:~:text=Hydrogen%20(Na%2B)%2C%20Sodium,with%20a%20valence%20of%20three.*

185. *https://www.webmd.com/osteoporosis/news/20161011/calcium-supplements-may-not-be-heart-healthy#1.*

186. *https://www.webmd.com/osteoporosis/calcium-supplements-tips#1.*

187. *https://www.usbr.gov/lc/phoenix/programs/cass/pdf/Phase2/3BSalinityControlWWTPAppendixB.pdf.*

188. Neal, J.B. and M. Neal, *Effect of hard water and MgSO4 on rabbit atherosclerosis.* Arch Pathol, 1962. **73**: p. 400-3.

189. *https://www.myfewa.com/hard-water-tampa.html.*

190. *https://phys.org/news/2014-06-science-coffee.html.*

191. *https://www.worldbaristachampionship.org/wp-content/uploads/2015/02/2014-WBC-RANKINGS.pdf?x58757.*

192. Chipperfield, B. and J.R. Chipperfield, *Magnesium and the heart.* Am Heart J, 1977. **93**(6): p. 679-82.

193. Heroux, O., D. Peter, and A. Tanner, *Effect of a chronic suboptimal intake of magnesium on magnesium and calcium content of bone and on bone strength of the rat.* Can J Physiol Pharmacol, 1975. **53**(2): p. 304-10.

194. Heroux, O., D. Peter, and A. Heggtveit, *Long-term effect of suboptimal dietary magnesium on magnesium and calcium contents of organs, on cold tolerance and on lifespan, and its pathological consequences in rats.* J Nutr, 1977. **107**(9): p. 1640-52.

195. Kubena, K.S. and J. Durlach, *Historical review of the effects of marginal intake of magnesium in chronic experimental magnesium deficiency.* Magnes Res, 1990. **3**(3): p. 219-26.

196. Lehr, D., R. Chau, and S. Irene, *Possible role of magnesium loss in the pathogenesis of myocardial fiber necrosis.* Recent Adv Stud Cardiac Struct Metab, 1975. **6**: p. 95-109.

197. Anderson, T.W., et al., *Letter: Water hardness and magnesium in heart muscle.* Lancet, 1973. **2**(7842): p. 1390-1.

198. Schwalfenberg, G.K. and S.J. Genuis, *The Importance of Magnesium in Clinical Healthcare.* Scientifica (Cairo), 2017. **2017**: p. 4179326.

199. *World Health Organization. Cardiovascular Diseases (CVDs). Retrieved from https://www.who.int/news-room/fact-sheets/detail/cardiovascular-diseases-(cvds).*

200. Birger, M., et al., *Spending on Cardiovascular Disease and Cardiovascular Risk Factors in the United States: 1996 to 2016.* Circulation, 2021. **144**(4): p. 271-282.

201. Tangvoraphonkchai, K. and A. Davenport, *Magnesium and Cardiovascular Disease.* Adv Chronic Kidney Dis, 2018. **25**(3): p. 251-260.

202. Severino, P., et al., *Prevention of Cardiovascular Disease: Screening for Magnesium Deficiency.* Cardiol Res Pract, 2019. **2019**: p. 4874921.

203. DiNicolantonio, J.J., J. Liu, and J.H. O'Keefe, *Magnesium for the prevention and treatment of cardiovascular disease.* Open Heart, 2018. **5**(2): p. e000775.

204. Rosique-Esteban, N., et al., *Dietary Magnesium and Cardiovascular Disease: A Review with Emphasis in Epidemiological Studies.* Nutrients, 2018. **10**(2).

205. Lichton, I.J., *Dietary intake levels and requirements of Mg and Ca for different segments of the U.S. population.* Magnesium, 1989. **8**(3-4): p. 117-23.

206. Shaper, A.G., *Soft water, heart attacks, and stroke.* Jama, 1974. **230**(1): p. 130-1.

207. Whang, R. and K.W. Ryder, *Frequency of hypomagnesemia and hypermagnesemia. Requested vs routine.* Jama, 1990. **263**(22): p. 3063-4.

208. Ryzen, E., U. Elkayam, and R.K. Rude, *Low blood mononuclear cell magnesium in intensive cardiac care unit patients.* Am Heart J, 1986. **111**(3): p. 475-80.

209. Reinhart, R.A., *Magnesium metabolism. A review with special reference to the relationship between intracellular content and serum levels.* Arch Intern Med, 1988. **148**(11): p. 2415-20.

210. Elin, R.J., *Status of the determination of magnesium in mononuclear blood cells in humans.* Magnesium, 1988. **7**(5-6): p. 300-5.

211. Purvis, J.R. and A. Movahed, *Magnesium disorders and cardiovascular diseases.* Clin Cardiol, 1992. **15**(8): p. 556-68.

212. Fischer, P.W. and A. Giroux, *Effects of dietary magnesium on sodium-potassium pump action in the heart of rats.* J Nutr, 1987. **117**(12): p. 2091-5.

213. Madden, J.A., et al., *Sodium kinetics and membrane potential in aorta of magnesium-deficient rats.* Magnesium, 1984. **3**(2): p. 73-80.

214. Sheehan, J.P. and M.S. Seelig, *Interactions of magnesium and potassium in the pathogenesis of cardiovascular disease.* Magnesium, 1984. **3**(4-6): p. 301-14.

215. Weglicki, W.B. and T.M. Phillips, *Pathobiology of magnesium deficiency: a cytokine/neurogenic inflammation hypothesis.* Am J Physiol, 1992. **263**(3 Pt 2): p. R734-7.

216. Zheltova, A.A., et al., *Magnesium deficiency and oxidative stress: an update.* Biomedicine (Taipei), 2016. **6**(4): p. 20.

217. Mazur, A., et al., *Magnesium and the inflammatory response: potential physiopathological implications.* Arch Biochem Biophys, 2007. **458**(1): p. 48-56.

218. *https://www.who.int/news-room/fact-sheets/detail/hypertension.*

219. *https://www.cdc.gov/bloodpressure/about.htm.*

220. Singh, R.B., et al., *Magnesium metabolism in essential hypertension.* Acta Cardiol, 1989. **44**(4): p. 313-22.

221. Altura, B.M. and B.T. Altura, *Interactions of Mg and K on blood vessels--aspects in view of hypertension. Review of present status and new findings.* Magnesium, 1984. **3**(4-6): p. 175-94.

222. Ryan, M.P. and H.R. Brady, *The role of magnesium in the prevention and control of hypertension.* Ann Clin Res, 1984. **16 Suppl 43**: p. 81-8.

223. Shibutani, Y., et al., *Serum and erythrocyte magnesium levels in junior high school students: relation to blood pressure and a family history of hypertension.* Magnesium, 1988. **7**(4): p. 188-94.

224. Maier, J.A., et al., *Low magnesium promotes endothelial cell dysfunction: implications for atherosclerosis, inflammation and thrombosis.* Biochim Biophys Acta, 2004. **1689**(1): p. 13-21.

225. Ferrè, S., et al., *Magnesium deficiency promotes a pro-atherogenic phenotype in cultured human endothelial cells via activation of NFkB*. Biochim Biophys Acta, 2010. **1802**(11): p. 952-8.

226. Shechter, M., *The role of magnesium as antithrombotic therapy*. Wien Med Wochenschr, 2000. **150**(15-16): p. 343-7.

227. Briel, R.C., T.H. Lippert, and H.P. Zahradnik, *[Changes in blood coagulation, thrombocyte function and vascular prostacyclin synthesis caused by magnesium sulfate]*. Geburtshilfe Frauenheilkd, 1987. **47**(5): p. 332-6.

228. Saito, K., et al., *Effects of oral magnesium on blood pressure and red cell sodium transport in patients receiving long-term thiazide diuretics for hypertension*. Am J Hypertens, 1988. **1**(3 Pt 3): p. 71s-74s.

229. Rayssiguier, Y. and E. Rock, *Commentary to the letter to the editor re: role of magnesium in metabolic syndrome*. Magnes Res, 2010. **23**(3): p. 146.

230. Zhang, X., et al., *Effects of Magnesium Supplementation on Blood Pressure: A Meta-Analysis of Randomized Double-Blind Placebo-Controlled Trials*. Hypertension, 2016. **68**(2): p. 324-33.

231. Hattori, K., et al., *Intracellular magnesium deficiency and effect of oral magnesium on blood pressure and red cell sodium transport in diuretic-treated hypertensive patients*. Jpn Circ J, 1988. **52**(11): p. 1249-56.

232. Rosanoff, A. and M.R. Plesset, *Oral magnesium supplements decrease high blood pressure (SBP>155 mmHg) in hypertensive subjects on anti-hypertensive medications: a targeted meta-analysis*. Magnes Res, 2013. **26**(3): p. 93-9.

233. Kass, L., J. Weekes, and L. Carpenter, *Effect of magnesium supplementation on blood pressure: a meta-analysis*. Eur J Clin Nutr, 2012. **66**(4): p. 411-8.

234. Rafieian-Kopaei, M., et al., *Atherosclerosis: process, indicators, risk factors and new hopes*. Int J Prev Med, 2014. **5**(8): p. 927-46.

235. Neels, J.G., G. Leftheriotis, and G. Chinetti, *Atherosclerosis Calcification: Focus on Lipoproteins*. Metabolites, 2023. **13**(3).

236. Roberti, A., L.E. Chaffey, and D.R. Greaves, *NF-κB Signaling and Inflammation-Drug Repurposing to Treat Inflammatory Disorders?* Biology (Basel), 2022. **11**(3).

237. Cancemi, P., et al., *The Role of Matrix Metalloproteinases (MMP-2 and MMP-9) in Ageing and Longevity: Focus on Sicilian Long-Living Individuals (LLIs)*. Mediators Inflamm, 2020. **2020**: p. 8635158.

238. Shah, N.C., et al., *Mg deficiency results in modulation of serum lipids, glutathione, and NO synthase isozyme activation in cardiovascular tissues: relevance to de novo synthesis of ceramide, serum Mg and atherogenesis*. Int J Clin Exp Med, 2011. **4**(2): p. 103-18.

239. Nakamura, M., et al., *DIETARY EFFECT OF MAGNESIUM ON CHOLESTEROL-INDUCED ATHEROSCLEROSIS OF RABBITS*. J Atheroscler Res, 1965. **5**(2): p. 145-58.

240. Rasmussen, H.S., et al., *Influence of magnesium substitution therapy on blood lipid composition in patients with ischemic heart disease. A double-blind, placebo controlled study*. Arch Intern Med, 1989. **149**(5): p. 1050-3.

241. Gupta, B.K., D. Glicklich, and V.A. Tellis, *Magnesium repletion therapy improved lipid metabolism in hypomagnesemic renal transplant recipients: a pilot study*. Transplantation, 1999. **67**(11): p. 1485-7.

242. Cojocaru, I.M., et al., *Serum magnesium in patients with acute ischemic stroke.* Rom J Intern Med, 2007. **45**(3): p. 269-73.

243. Stendig-Lindberg, G., *Sudden death of athletes: is it due to long-term changes in serum magnesium, lipids and blood sugar?* J Basic Clin Physiol Pharmacol, 1992. **3**(2): p. 153-64.

244. *https://my.clevelandclinic.org/health/diseases/16841-cardiomyopathy.*

245. Ahmad, A. and S. Bloom, *Sodium pump and calcium channel modulation of Mg-deficiency cardiomyopathy.* Am J Cardiovasc Pathol, 1989. **2**(4): p. 277-83.

246. Herbaczynska-Cedro, K. and B. Gajkowska, *Effect of magnesium on myocardial damage induced by epinephrine. Ultrastructural and cytochemical study.* Cardioscience, 1992. **3**(3): p. 197-203.

247. Giles, T.D., B.J. Iteld, and K.L. Rives, *The cardiomyopathy of hypoparathyroidism. Another reversible form of heart muscle disease.* Chest, 1981. **79**(2): p. 225-9.

248. *Seelig MS. Magnesium deficiency in the pathogenesis of disease: early roots of cardiovascular skeletal, and renal abnormalities, 1980.*

249. Valiathan, M.S., et al., *A geochemical basis for endomyocardial fibrosis.* Cardiovasc Res, 1989. **23**(7): p. 647-8.

250. Valiathan, S.M. and C.C. Kartha, *Endomyocardial fibrosis--the possible connexion with myocardial levels of magnesium and cerium.* Int J Cardiol, 1990. **28**(1): p. 1-5.

251. *Congestive heart failure: Prevention, treatment and research. Johns Hopkins Medicine. (2022, April 8). https://www.hopkinsmedicine.org/health/conditions-and-diseases/congestive-heart-failure-prevention-treatment-and-research.*

252. *World Health Organization. (n.d.). Cardiovascular diseases (cvds). World Health Organization. https://www.who.int/news-room/fact-sheets/detail/cardiovascular-diseases-(cvds).*

253. Gottlieb, S.S., *Importance of magnesium in congestive heart failure.* Am J Cardiol, 1989. **63**(14): p. 39g-42g.

254. Wester, P.O. and T. Dyckner, *Intracellular electrolytes in cardiac failure.* Acta Med Scand Suppl, 1986. **707**: p. 33-6.

255. Song, E.K. and S.M. Kang, *Micronutrient Deficiency Independently Predicts Adverse Health Outcomes in Patients With Heart Failure.* J Cardiovasc Nurs, 2017. **32**(1): p. 47-53.

256. Bashir, Y., et al., *Effects of long-term oral magnesium chloride replacement in congestive heart failure secondary to coronary artery disease.* Am J Cardiol, 1993. **72**(15): p. 1156-62.

257. Stepura, O.B. and A.I. Martynow, *Magnesium orotate in severe congestive heart failure (MACH).* Int J Cardiol, 2009. **131**(2): p. 293-5.

258. Ralston, M.A., et al., *Magnesium content of serum, circulating mononuclear cells, skeletal muscle, and myocardium in congestive heart failure.* Circulation, 1989. **80**(3): p. 573-80.

259. *professional, C. C. medical. (n.d.). What you need to know about arrhythmias. Cleveland Clinic. https://my.clevelandclinic.org/health/diseases/16749-arrhythmia.*

260. Cohen, L., A. Laor, and R. Kitzes, *Prolonged Q-Tc interval and decreased lymphocyte magnesium in congestive heart failure.* Magnesium, 1984. **3**(3): p. 164-8.

261. Davis, W.H. and F. Ziady, *The effect of oral magnesium chloride therapy on the QTc and QUc intervals of the electrocardiogram.* S Afr Med J, 1978. **53**(15): p. 591-3.

262. Laban, E. and G.A. Charbon, *Magnesium and cardiac arrhythmias: nutrient or drug?* J Am Coll Nutr, 1986. **5**(6): p. 521-32.

263.*St-segment   depression   and   T-Wave   Inversion.   (n.d.-a).https://www.ccjm.org/content/ccjom/78/6/404.full.pdf.*

264. Boyd, J.C., et al., *Relationship of potassium and magnesium concentrations in serum to cardiac arrhythmias.* Clin Chem, 1984. **30**(5): p. 754-7.

265. Dyckner, T. and P.O. Wester, *Potassium/magnesium depletion in patients with cardiovascular disease.* Am J Med, 1987. **82**(3a): p. 11-7.

266. Hollifield, J.W., *Thiazide treatment of hypertension. Effects of thiazide diuretics on serum potassium, magnesium, and ventricular ectopy.* Am J Med, 1986. **80**(4a): p. 8-12.

267. Hollifield, J.W., *Potassium and magnesium abnormalities: diuretics and arrhythmias in hypertension.* Am J Med, 1984. **77**(5a): p. 28-32.

268. Dyckner, T. and P.O. Wester, *Relation between potassium, magnesium and cardiac arrhythmias.* Acta Med Scand Suppl, 1981. **647**: p. 163-9.

269. Dyckner, T. and P.O. Wester, *Ventricular extrasystoles and intracellular electrolytes before and after potassium and magnesium infusions in patients on diuretic treatment.* Am Heart J, 1979. **97**(1): p. 12-8.

270. Cannon, L.A., et al., *Magnesium levels in cardiac arrest victims: relationship between magnesium levels and successful resuscitation.* Ann Emerg Med, 1987. **16**(11): p. 1195-9.

271. *Patti L, Ashurst JV. Supraventricular Tachycardia. [Updated 2023 Aug 7]. In: StatPearls [Internet]. Treasure Island (FL): StatPearls Publishing; 2024 Jan-. Available from: https://www.ncbi.nlm.nih.gov/books/NBK441972/.*

272. Ganga, H.V., et al., *Magnesium adjunctive therapy in atrial arrhythmias.* Pacing Clin Electrophysiol, 2013. **36**(10): p. 1308-18.

273. Maurat, J.P., et al., *[Cardiovascular pathology and magnesium].* Therapie, 1993. **48**(6): p. 599-607.

274. Khan, A.M., et al., *Low serum magnesium and the development of atrial fibrillation in the community: the Framingham Heart Study.* Circulation, 2013. **127**(1): p. 33-8.

275. DeCarli, C., G. Sprouse, and J.C. LaRosa, *Serum magnesium levels in symptomatic atrial fibrillation and their relation to rhythm control by intravenous digoxin.* Am J Cardiol, 1986. **57**(11): p. 956-9.

276. Lewis, R.V., et al., *Oral magnesium reduces ventricular ectopy in digitalised patients with chronic atrial fibrillation.* Eur J Clin Pharmacol, 1990. **38**(2): p. 107-10.

277. Cohen, L. and R. Kitzes, *Magnesium sulfate and digitalis-toxic arrhythmias.* Jama, 1983. **249**(20): p. 2808-10.

278. *Foth C, Gangwani MK, Ahmed I, et al. Ventricular Tachycardia. [Updated 2023 Jul 30]. In: StatPearls [Internet]. Treasure Island (FL): StatPearls Publishing; 2024 Jan-. Available from: https://www.ncbi.nlm.nih.gov/books/NBK532954/.*

279. Iseri, L.T., *Role of magnesium in cardiac tachyarrhythmias.* Am J Cardiol, 1990. **65**(23): p. 47k-50k.

280. Bean, B.L. and P.J. Varghese, *Role of dietary magnesium deficiency in the pressor and arrhythmogenic response to epinephrine in the intact dog.* Am Heart J, 1994. **127**(1): p. 96-102.

281. Krasner, B.S., R. Girdwood, and H. Smith, *The effect of slow releasing oral magnesium chloride on the QTc interval of the electrocardiogram during open heart surgery.* Can Anaesth Soc J, 1981. **28**(4): p. 329-33.

282. Raghu, C., P. Peddeswara Rao, and D. Seshagiri Rao, *Protective effect of intravenous magnesium in acute myocardial infarction following thrombolytic therapy.* Int J Cardiol, 1999. **71**(3): p. 209-15.

283. Papaceit, J., et al., *[Severe heart arrhythmia secondary to magnesium depletion. Torsade de pointes].* Rev Esp Anestesiol Reanim, 1990. **37**(1): p. 28-31.

284. *Mayo Foundation for Medical Education and Research. (2023, January 19). Sudden cardiac arrest. Mayo Clinic. https://www.mayoclinic.org/diseases-conditions/sudden-cardiac-arrest/symptoms-causes/syc20350634#:~:text=The%20most%20common%20cause%20of,uselessly%20instead%20of%20pumping%20blood.*

285. *Tseng ZH, Salazar JW, Olgin JE, Ursell PC, Kim AS, Bedigian A, Probert J, Hart AP, Moffatt E, Vittinghoff E. Refining the World Health Organization Definition: Predicting Autopsy-Defined Sudden Arrhythmic Deaths Among Presumed Sudden Cardiac Deaths in the POST SCD Study. Circ Arrhythm Electrophysiol. 2019 Jul;12(7):e007171. doi: 10.1161/CIRCEP.119.007171. Epub 2019 Jun 28. PMID: 31248279; PMCID: PMC6738572.*

286. Eisenberg, M.J., *Magnesium deficiency and sudden death.* Am Heart J, 1992. **124**(2): p. 544-9.

287. Singh, R.B., V.P. Singh, and E.A. Cameron, *Magnesium in atherosclerotic cardiovascular disease and sudden death.* Acta Cardiol, 1981. **36**(6): p. 411-29.

288. Altura, B.M., et al., *Hypomagnesemia and vasoconstriction: possible relationship to etiology of sudden death ischemic heart disease and hypertensive vascular diseases.* Artery, 1981. **9**(3): p. 212-31.

289. Turlapaty, P.D. and B.M. Altura, *Magnesium deficiency produces spasms of coronary arteries: relationship to etiology of sudden death ischemic heart disease.* Science, 1980. **208**(4440): p. 198-200.

290. Altura, B.M., *Sudden-death ischemic heart disease and dietary magnesium intake: is the target site coronary vascular smooth muscle?* Med Hypotheses, 1979. **5**(8): p. 843-8.

291. *Swarup S, Patibandla S, Grossman SA. Coronary Artery Vasospasm. [Updated 2023 Jul 4]. In: StatPearls [Internet]. Treasure Island (FL): StatPearls Publishing; 2024 Jan-. Available from: https://www.ncbi.nlm.nih.gov/books/NBK470181/#.*

292. *Chadda KD, Schultz NA. Magnesium deficiency and coronary vasospasm: role in sudden cardiac death. Magnesium 1982;1:86–94.*

293. Yanagisawa-Miwa, A., H. Ito, and T. Sugimoto, *Effects of insulin on vasoconstriction induced by thromboxane A2 in porcine coronary artery.* Circulation, 1990. **81**(5): p. 1654-9.

294. Tanabe, K., et al., *Variant angina due to deficiency of intracellular magnesium.* Clin Cardiol, 1990. **13**(9): p. 663-5.

295. Guo, H., et al., *Relationship between the degree of intracellular magnesium deficiency and the frequency of chest pain in women with variant angina.* Herz, 2004. **29**(3): p. 299-303.

296. Teragawa, H., et al., *The preventive effect of magnesium on coronary spasm in patients with vasospastic angina.* Chest, 2000. **118**(6): p. 1690-5.

297. *Thrombosis: What you need to know. Cleveland Clinic. https://my.clevelandclinic.org/health/diseases/22242-thrombosis.*

298. Parsons RS, Butler T, Sellars EP. *The treatment of coronary artery disease with parenteral magnesium sulphate.* Med Proc 1959:487.

299. Jeppesen, B.B., *Magnesium status in patients with acute myocardial infarction: a pilot study.* Magnesium, 1986. **5**(2): p. 95-100.

300. Cantón, R., et al., *In vitro and in vivo antiaggregant effects of magnesium halogenates.* Thromb Haemost, 1987. **58**(4): p. 957-9.

301. Lox, C.D., M.M. Dorsett, and R.M. Hampton, *Observations on clotting activity during pre-eclampsia.* Clin Exp Hypertens B, 1983. **2**(2): p. 179-90.

302. Paolisso, G., et al., *Magnesium administration reduces platelet hyperaggregability in NIDDM.* Diabetes Care, 1989. **12**(2): p. 167-8.

303. *Problem: Mitral valve prolapse.* www.heart.org. (2023, October 19). https://www.heart.org/en/health-topics/heart-valve-problems-and-disease/heart-valve-problems-and-causes/problem-mitral-valve-prolapse.

304. Kitliński, M., et al., *Is magnesium deficit in lymphocytes a part of the mitral valve prolapse syndrome?* Magnes Res, 2004. **17**(1): p. 39-45.

305. Lichodziejewska, B., et al., *Clinical symptoms of mitral valve prolapse are related to hypomagnesemia and attenuated by magnesium supplementation.* Am J Cardiol, 1997. **79**(6): p. 768-72.

306. *World Health Organization.* (n.d.). World Health Organization. https://www.emro.who.int/health-topics/stroke-cerebrovascular-accident/index.html.

307. *Global stroke fact sheet 2022.* (n.d.-a). https://www.worldstroke.org/assets/downloads/WSO_Global_Stroke_Fact_Sheet.pdf.

308. Szabó C, Hardebo JE, Salford LG. *Role of endothelium in the responses of human intracranial arteries to a slight reduction of extracellular magnesium.* Exp Physiol 1992;77:209–11.

309. Amighi, J., et al., *Low serum magnesium predicts neurological events in patients with advanced atherosclerosis.* Stroke, 2004. **35**(1): p. 22-7.

310. Pizzino, G., et al., *Oxidative Stress: Harms and Benefits for Human Health.* Oxid Med Cell Longev, 2017. **2017**: p. 8416763.

311. Wiles, M.E., T.L. Wagner, and W.B. Weglicki, *Effect of acute magnesium deficiency (MgD) on aortic endothelial cell (EC) oxidant production.* Life Sci, 1997. **60**(3): p. 221-36.

312. Kumar, B.P. and K. Shivakumar, *Depressed antioxidant defense in rat heart in experimental magnesium deficiency. Implications for the pathogenesis of myocardial lesions.* Biol Trace Elem Res, 1997. **60**(1-2): p. 139-44.

313. Hans, C.P., D.P. Chaudhary, and D.D. Bansal, *Magnesium deficiency increases oxidative stress in rats.* Indian J Exp Biol, 2002. **40**(11): p. 1275-9.

314. Freedman, A.M., M.M. Cassidy, and W.B. Weglicki, *Magnesium-deficient myocardium demonstrates an increased susceptibility to an in vivo oxidative stress.* Magnes Res, 1991. **4**(3-4): p. 185-9.

315. Kharb, S. and V. Singh, *Magnesium deficiency potentiates free radical production associated with myocardial infarction.* J Assoc Physicians India, 2000. **48**(5): p. 484-5.

316. Urdal, P., K. Landmark, and G.M. Basmo, *Mononuclear cell magnesium and retention of magnesium after intravenous loading in patients with acute myocardial infarction.* Scand J Clin Lab Invest, 1992. **52**(7): p. 763-6.

317. Rasmussen, H.S., et al., *Magnesium deficiency in patients with ischemic heart disease with and without acute myocardial infarction uncovered by an intravenous loading test.* Arch Intern Med, 1988. **148**(2): p. 329-32.

318. *Maurat JP, Kantelip JP, Anguenot T, et al. [Cardiovascular pathology and magnesium]. Therapie 1993;48:599–607.*

319. Cheng, C.H., L.R. Chen, and K.H. Chen, *Osteoporosis Due to Hormone Imbalance: An Overview of the Effects of Estrogen Deficiency and Glucocorticoid Overuse on Bone Turnover.* Int J Mol Sci, 2022. **23**(3).

320. Bolland, M.J., et al., *Calcium supplements with or without vitamin D and risk of cardiovascular events: reanalysis of the Women's Health Initiative limited access dataset and meta-analysis.* Bmj, 2011. **342**: p. d2040.

321. Xiao, Q., et al., *Dietary and supplemental calcium intake and cardiovascular disease mortality: the National Institutes of Health-AARP diet and health study.* JAMA Intern Med, 2013. **173**(8): p. 639-46.

322. Li, K., et al., *Associations of dietary calcium intake and calcium supplementation with myocardial infarction and stroke risk and overall cardiovascular mortality in the Heidelberg cohort of the European Prospective Investigation into Cancer and Nutrition study (EPIC-Heidelberg).* Heart, 2012. **98**(12): p. 920-5.

323. Anderson, J.J., et al., *Calcium Intake From Diet and Supplements and the Risk of Coronary Artery Calcification and its Progression Among Older Adults: 10-Year Follow-up of the Multi-Ethnic Study of Atherosclerosis (MESA).* J Am Heart Assoc, 2016. **5**(10).

324. Wang, L., J.E. Manson, and H.D. Sesso, *Calcium intake and risk of cardiovascular disease: a review of prospective studies and randomized clinical trials.* Am J Cardiovasc Drugs, 2012. **12**(2): p. 105-16.

325. Anderson, J.L., et al., *Parathyroid hormone, vitamin D, renal dysfunction, and cardiovascular disease: dependent or independent risk factors?* Am Heart J, 2011. **162**(2): p. 331-339.e2.

326. Peiris, A.N., D. Youssef, and W.B. Grant, *Secondary hyperparathyroidism: benign bystander or culpable contributor to adverse health outcomes?* South Med J, 2012. **105**(1): p. 36-42.

327. Ellam, T.J. and T.J. Chico, *Phosphate: the new cholesterol? The role of the phosphate axis in non-uremic vascular disease.* Atherosclerosis, 2012. **220**(2): p. 310-8.

328. Samelson, E.J., et al., *Calcium intake is not associated with increased coronary artery calcification: the Framingham Study.* Am J Clin Nutr, 2012. **96**(6): p. 1274-80.

329. Burt, M.G., et al., *Acute effect of calcium citrate on serum calcium and cardiovascular function.* J Bone Miner Res, 2013. **28**(2): p. 412-8.

330. Bhattacharya, R.K., *Does widespread calcium supplementation pose cardiovascular risk? No: concerns are unwarranted.* Am Fam Physician, 2013. **87**(3): p. Online.

331. Lewis, J.R., et al., *Calcium supplementation and the risks of atherosclerotic vascular disease in older women: results of a 5-year RCT and a 4.5-year follow-up.* J Bone Miner Res, 2011. **26**(1): p. 35-41.

332. Zhang, W., et al., *Associations of dietary magnesium intake with mortality from cardiovascular disease: the JACC study.* Atherosclerosis, 2012. **221**(2): p. 587-95.

333. Lee, S.Y., et al., *Low serum magnesium is associated with coronary artery calcification in a Korean population at low risk for cardiovascular disease.* Nutr Metab Cardiovasc Dis, 2015. **25**(11): p. 1056-61.

334. Pokan, R., et al., *Oral magnesium therapy, exercise heart rate, exercise tolerance, and myocardial function in coronary artery disease patients.* Br J Sports Med, 2006. **40**(9): p. 773-8.

335. Shechter, M., *Magnesium and cardiovascular system.* Magnes Res, 2010. **23**(2): p. 60-72.

336. Shechter, M., et al., *Oral magnesium supplementation inhibits platelet-dependent thrombosis in patients with coronary artery disease.* Am J Cardiol, 1999. **84**(2): p. 152-6.

337. Shechter, M., et al., *Oral magnesium therapy improves endothelial function in patients with coronary artery disease.* Circulation, 2000. **102**(19): p. 2353-8.

338. Grabarek, Z., *Insights into modulation of calcium signaling by magnesium in calmodulin, troponin C and related EF-hand proteins.* Biochim Biophys Acta, 2011. **1813**(5): p. 913-21.

339. Malmendal, A., et al., *Battle for the EF-hands: magnesium-calcium interference in calmodulin.* Biochemistry, 1999. **38**(36): p. 11844-50.

340. Iseri, L.T. and J.H. French, *Magnesium: nature's physiologic calcium blocker.* Am Heart J, 1984. **108**(1): p. 188-93.

341. Massy, Z.A. and T.B. Drüeke, *Magnesium and outcomes in patients with chronic kidney disease: focus on vascular calcification, atherosclerosis and survival.* Clin Kidney J, 2012. **5**(Suppl 1): p. i52-i61.

342. Hruby, A., et al., *Magnesium intake is inversely associated with coronary artery calcification: the Framingham Heart Study.* JACC Cardiovasc Imaging, 2014. **7**(1): p. 59-69.

343. Maier, J.A.M., et al., *Magnesium and the Brain: A Focus on Neuroinflammation and Neurodegeneration.* Int J Mol Sci, 2022. **24**(1).

344. Kirkland, A.E., G.L. Sarlo, and K.F. Holton, *The Role of Magnesium in Neurological Disorders.* Nutrients, 2018. **10**(6).

345. Bhaskar, S., D. Hemavathy, and S. Prasad, *Prevalence of chronic insomnia in adult patients and its correlation with medical comorbidities.* J Family Med Prim Care, 2016. **5**(4): p. 780-784.

346. Holder, S. and N.S. Narula, *Common Sleep Disorders in Adults: Diagnosis and Management.* Am Fam Physician, 2022. **105**(4): p. 397-405.

347. Cuciureanu MD, Vink R. Magnesium and stress. In: Vink R, Nechifor M, editors. *Magnesium in the Central Nervous System [Internet].* Adelaide (AU): University of Adelaide Press; 2011. Available from: https://www.ncbi.nlm.nih.gov/books/NBK507250/.

348. Arab, A., et al., *The Role of Magnesium in Sleep Health: a Systematic Review of Available Literature.* Biol Trace Elem Res, 2023. **201**(1): p. 121-128.

349. U.S. Department of Health and Human Services. (n.d.). What is insomnia?. National Heart Lung and Blood Institute. https://www.nhlbi.nih.gov/health/insomnia.

350. Abbasi, B., et al., *The effect of magnesium supplementation on primary insomnia in elderly: A double-blind placebo-controlled clinical trial.* J Res Med Sci, 2012. **17**(12): p. 1161-9.

351. Dominguez, L.J., N. Veronese, and M. Barbagallo, *Magnesium and the Hallmarks of Aging.* Nutrients, 2024. **16**(4).

352. Boyle, N.B., C. Lawton, and L. Dye, *The Effects of Magnesium Supplementation on Subjective Anxiety and Stress-A Systematic Review.* Nutrients, 2017. **9**(5).

353. Nielsen, F.H., *Magnesium deficiency and increased inflammation: current perspectives.* J Inflamm Res, 2018. **11**: p. 25-34.

354. Nielsen, F.H., L.K. Johnson, and H. Zeng, *Magnesium supplementation improves indicators of low magnesium status and inflammatory stress in adults older than 51 years with poor quality sleep.* Magnes Res, 2010. **23**(4): p. 158-68.

355. Djokic, G., et al., *The Effects of Magnesium - Melatonin - Vit B Complex Supplementation in Treatment of Insomnia.* Open Access Maced J Med Sci, 2019. **7**(18): p. 3101-3105.

356. Billyard, A.J., D.L. Eggett, and K.B. Franz, *Dietary magnesium deficiency decreases plasma melatonin in rats.* Magnes Res, 2006. **19**(3): p. 157-61.

357. Depoortere, H., D. Françon, and J. Llopis, *Effects of a magnesium-deficient diet on sleep organization in rats.* Neuropsychobiology, 1993. **27**(4): p. 237-45.

358. *Home - restless legs syndrome foundation (no date) Home - Restless Legs Syndrome Foundation. Available at: https://www.rls.org/ (Accessed: 02 May 2024).*

359. *Mansur A, Castillo PR, Rocha Cabrero F, et al. Restless Legs Syndrome. [Updated 2023 Feb 27]. In: StatPearls [Internet]. Treasure Island (FL): StatPearls Publishing; 2024 Jan-. Available from: https://www.ncbi.nlm.nih.gov/books/NBK430878/.*

360. Hornyak, M., et al., *Magnesium therapy for periodic leg movements-related insomnia and restless legs syndrome: an open pilot study.* Sleep, 1998. **21**(5): p. 501-5.

361. Popoviciu, L., et al., *Clinical, EEG, electromyographic and polysomnographic studies in restless legs syndrome caused by magnesium deficiency.* Rom J Neurol Psychiatry, 1993. **31**(1): p. 55-61.

362. *Slowik JM, Sankari A, Collen JF. Obstructive Sleep Apnea. [Updated 2022 Dec 11]. In: StatPearls [Internet]. Treasure Island (FL): StatPearls Publishing; 2024 Jan-. Available from: https://www.ncbi.nlm.nih.gov/books/NBK459252/.*

363. Al Wadee, Z., S.L. Ooi, and S.C. Pak, *Serum Magnesium Levels in Patients with Obstructive Sleep Apnoea: A Systematic Review and Meta-Analysis.* Biomedicines, 2022. **10**(9).

364. Liu, M. and S.C. Dudley, Jr., *Magnesium, Oxidative Stress, Inflammation, and Cardiovascular Disease.* Antioxidants (Basel), 2020. **9**(10).

365. *Sekhon S, Gupta V. Mood Disorder. [Updated 2023 May 8]. In: StatPearls [Internet]. Treasure Island (FL): StatPearls Publishing; 2024 Jan-. Available from: https://www.ncbi.nlm.nih.gov/books/NBK558911/.*

366. *Most common mood disorders: How many mood disorders are there? (2023) The Recovery Village Drug and Alcohol Rehab. Available at: https://www.therecoveryvillage.com/mental-health/mood-disorders/mood-disorders-statistics/ (Accessed: 25 April 2024).*

367. *Biederman J. (2005). Attention-deficit/hyperactivity disorder: a selective overview. Biological psychiatry, 57(11), 1215–1220. https://doi.org/10.1016/j.biopsych.2004.10.020.*

368. *Mental disorders (no date) World Health Organization. Available at: https://www.who.int/news-room/fact-sheets/detail/mental-disorders (Accessed: 25 April 2024).*

369. *Depressive disorder (depression) (no date) World Health Organization. Available at: https://www.who.int/news-room/fact-sheets/detail/depression (Accessed: 25 April 2024).*

370. Phelan, D., et al., *Magnesium and mood disorders: systematic review and meta-analysis.* BJPsych Open, 2018. **4**(4): p. 167-179.

371. *World Health Organization. (n.d.). Anxiety disorders. World Health Organization. https://www.who.int/news-room/fact-sheets/detail/anxiety-disorders.*

372. *(2024) The American Institute of Stress. Available at: https://www.stress.org/ (Accessed: 21 April 2024).*

373. *American Psychological Association. (n.d.). How stress affects your health. American Psychological Association. https://www.apa.org/topics/stress/health.*

374. Tarasov, E.A., et al., *[Magnesium deficiency and stress: Issues of their relationship, diagnostic tests, and approaches to therapy].* Ter Arkh, 2015. **87**(9): p. 114-122.

375. Cuciureanu, M.D. and R. Vink, *Magnesium and stress*, in *Magnesium in the Central Nervous System*, R. Vink and M. Nechifor, Editors. 2011, University of Adelaide Press

© 2011 The Authors.: Adelaide (AU).

376. Murck, H., *Magnesium and affective disorders.* Nutr Neurosci, 2002. **5**(6): p. 375-89.

377. Whyte, K.F., et al., *Adrenergic control of plasma magnesium in man.* Clin Sci (Lond), 1987. **72**(1): p. 135-8.

378. Cernak, I., et al., *Alterations in magnesium and oxidative status during chronic emotional stress.* Magnes Res, 2000. **13**(1): p. 29-36.

379. Grases, G., et al., *Anxiety and stress among science students. Study of calcium and magnesium alterations.* Magnes Res, 2006. **19**(2): p. 102-6.

380. Mocci, F., et al., *The effect of noise on serum and urinary magnesium and catecholamines in humans.* Occup Med (Lond), 2001. **51**(1): p. 56-61.

381. *Young E.A., Abelson J.L., Liberzon I. Stress hormones and anxiety disorders. In: Blanchard R.J., Blanchard D.C., Griebel G., Nutt D., editors. Handbook of Anxiety and Fear. Academic Press; Oxford: 2008. pp. 455–473.*

382. Lowry, C.A. and F.L. Moore, *Regulation of behavioral responses by corticotropin-releasing factor.* Gen Comp Endocrinol, 2006. **146**(1): p. 19-27.

383. *Charney D.S., Drevets W.C. Neurobiological basis of anxiety disorders. In: Davis K.L., Charney D., Coyle J.T., Nemeroff C., editors. Neuropsychopharmacology – 5th Generation of Progress. American College of Neuropsychopharmacology; Nashville: 2008.*

384. Sartori, S.B., et al., *Magnesium deficiency induces anxiety and HPA axis dysregulation: modulation by therapeutic drug treatment.* Neuropharmacology, 2012. **62**(1): p. 304-12.

385. Kumar, A., et al., *Gut Microbiota in Anxiety and Depression: Unveiling the Relationships and Management Options.* Pharmaceuticals (Basel), 2023. **16**(4).

386. Pyndt Jørgensen, B., et al., *Dietary magnesium deficiency affects gut microbiota and anxiety-like behaviour in C57BL/6N mice.* Acta Neuropsychiatr, 2015. **27**(5): p. 307-11.

387. *Akarachkova E. The role of magnesium deficiency in the formation of clinical manifestation of stress in women. Probl. Women Health. 2013;8:57.*

388. Noah, L., et al., *Impact of magnesium supplementation, in combination with vitamin B6, on stress and magnesium status: secondary data from a randomized controlled trial.* Magnes Res, 2020. **33**(3): p. 45-57.

389. Eby, G.A., 3rd and K.L. Eby, *Magnesium for treatment-resistant depression: a review and hypothesis.* Med Hypotheses, 2010. **74**(4): p. 649-60.

390. *Cuciureanu M., Vink R. Magnesium and stress. In: Vink R., Nechifor M., editors. Magnesium in the Central Nervous System. University of Adelaide Press; Adelaide, Australia: 2011.*

391. Schutten, J.C., et al., *Long-term magnesium supplementation improves glucocorticoid metabolism: A post-hoc analysis of an intervention trial.* Clin Endocrinol (Oxf), 2021. **94**(2): p. 150-157.

392. Zogović D., Pesić V., Dmitrasinović G., Dajak M., Plećas B., Batinić B., Popović D., Ignjatović S. *Pituitary-gonadal, pituitary-adrenocortical hormonal and IL-6 levels following long-term magnesium supplementation in male students. J. Med. Biochem. 2014;33:291–298. doi: 10.2478/jomb-2014-0016.*

393. Wienecke, E. and C. Nolden, *[Long-term HRV analysis shows stress reduction by magnesium intake].* MMW Fortschr Med, 2016. **158**(Suppl 6): p. 12-16.

394. Kim, H.G., et al., *Stress and Heart Rate Variability: A Meta-Analysis and Review of the Literature.* Psychiatry Investig, 2018. **15**(3): p. 235-245.

395. Pouteau, E., et al., *Superiority of magnesium and vitamin B6 over magnesium alone on severe stress in healthy adults with low magnesemia: A randomized, single-blind clinical trial.* PLoS One, 2018. **13**(12): p. e0208454.

396. *World Health Organization. (n.d.-b). Depressive disorder (depression). World Health Organization. https://www.who.int/news-room/fact-sheets/detail/depression.*

397. Moabedi, M., et al., *Magnesium supplementation beneficially affects depression in adults with depressive disorder: a systematic review and meta-analysis of randomized clinical trials.* Front Psychiatry, 2023. **14**: p. 1333261.

398. Cartwright, C., et al., *Long-term antidepressant use: patient perspectives of benefits and adverse effects.* Patient Prefer Adherence, 2016. **10**: p. 1401-7.

399. Szewczyk, B., et al., *Antidepressant activity of zinc and magnesium in view of the current hypotheses of antidepressant action.* Pharmacol Rep, 2008. **60**(5): p. 588-9.

400. Miranda, M., et al., *Brain-Derived Neurotrophic Factor: A Key Molecule for Memory in the Healthy and the Pathological Brain.* Front Cell Neurosci, 2019. **13**: p. 363.

401. Bathina, S. and U.N. Das, *Brain-derived neurotrophic factor and its clinical implications.* Arch Med Sci, 2015. **11**(6): p. 1164-78.

402. Serefko, A., et al., *Magnesium in depression.* Pharmacol Rep, 2013. **65**(3): p. 547-54.

403. Poleszak, E., et al., *NMDA/glutamate mechanism of antidepressant-like action of magnesium in forced swim test in mice.* Pharmacol Biochem Behav, 2007. **88**(2): p. 158-64.

404. Liu, Y.Z., Y.X. Wang, and C.L. Jiang, *Inflammation: The Common Pathway of Stress-Related Diseases.* Front Hum Neurosci, 2017. **11**: p. 316.

405. Chu A, Wadhwa R. *Selective Serotonin Reuptake Inhibitors. [Updated 2023 May 1]. In: StatPearls [Internet]. Treasure Island (FL): StatPearls Publishing; 2024 Jan-. Available from: https://www.ncbi.nlm.nih.gov/books/NBK554406/.*

406. Poleszak, E., *Modulation of antidepressant-like activity of magnesium by serotonergic system.* J Neural Transm (Vienna), 2007. **114**(9): p. 1129-34.

407. Samad, N., F. Yasmin, and N. Manzoor, *Biomarkers in Drug Free Subjects with Depression : Correlation with Tryptophan.* Psychiatry Investig, 2019. **16**(12): p. 948-953.

408. Islam, M.R., et al., *Alterations of serum macro-minerals and trace elements are associated with major depressive disorder: a case-control study.* BMC Psychiatry, 2018. **18**(1): p. 94.

409. Tarleton, E.K., et al., *The Association between Serum Magnesium Levels and Depression in an Adult Primary Care Population.* Nutrients, 2019. **11**(7).

410. Camardese, G., et al., *Plasma magnesium levels and treatment outcome in depressed patients.* Nutr Neurosci, 2012. **15**(2): p. 78-84.

411. Barragán-Rodríguez, L., M. Rodríguez-Morán, and F. Guerrero-Romero, *Efficacy and safety of oral magnesium supplementation in the treatment of depression in the elderly with type 2 diabetes: a randomized, equivalent trial.* Magnes Res, 2008. **21**(4): p. 218-23.

412. Eby, G.A., K.L. Eby, and H. Murk, *Magnesium and major depression*, in *Magnesium in the Central Nervous System*, R. Vink and M. Nechifor, Editors. 2011, University of Adelaide Press

© 2011 The Authors.: Adelaide (AU).

413. *Mughal S, Azhar Y, Siddiqui W. Postpartum Depression. [Updated 2022 Oct 7]. In: StatPearls [Internet]. Treasure Island (FL): StatPearls Publishing; 2024 Jan-. Available from: https://www.ncbi.nlm.nih.gov/books/NBK519070/.*

414. Etebary, S., et al., *Postpartum depression and role of serum trace elements.* Iran J Psychiatry, 2010. **5**(2): p. 40-6.

415. Winther, G., et al., *Dietary magnesium deficiency alters gut microbiota and leads to depressive-like behaviour.* Acta Neuropsychiatr, 2015. **27**(3): p. 168-76.

416. Afsharfar, M., et al., *The effects of magnesium supplementation on serum level of brain derived neurotrophic factor (BDNF) and depression status in patients with depression.* Clin Nutr ESPEN, 2021. **42**: p. 381-386.

417. Tarleton, E.K., et al., *Role of magnesium supplementation in the treatment of depression: A randomized clinical trial.* PLoS One, 2017. **12**(6): p. e0180067.

418. Eby, G.A. and K.L. Eby, *Rapid recovery from major depression using magnesium treatment.* Med Hypotheses, 2006. **67**(2): p. 362-70.

419. Wang, J., et al., *Zinc, Magnesium, Selenium and Depression: A Review of the Evidence, Potential Mechanisms and Implications.* Nutrients, 2018. **10**(5).

420. Shakya, P.R., et al., *Association between dietary patterns and adult depression symptoms based on principal component analysis, reduced-rank regression and partial least-squares.* Clin Nutr, 2020. **39**(9): p. 2811-2823.

421. Jacka, F.N., et al., *Association between magnesium intake and depression and anxiety in community-dwelling adults: the Hordaland Health Study.* Aust N Z J Psychiatry, 2009. **43**(1): p. 45-52.

422. *What are bipolar disorders?. Psychiatry.org - What Are Bipolar Disorders? (n.d.). https://www.psychiatry.org/patients-families/bipolar-disorders/what-are-bipolar-disorders.*

423. *U.S. Department of Health and Human Services. (n.d.). Bipolar disorder. National Institute of Mental Health. https://www.nimh.nih.gov/health/topics/bipolar-disorder.*

424. el-Beheiry, H. and E. Puil, *Effects of hypomagnesia on transmitter actions in neocortical slices.* Br J Pharmacol, 1990. **101**(4): p. 1006-10.

425. Oquendo, M.A., et al., *Brain serotonin transporter binding in depressed patients with bipolar disorder using positron emission tomography.* Arch Gen Psychiatry, 2007. **64**(2): p. 201-8.

426. Nechifor, M., *Magnesium in psychoses (schizophrenia and bipolar disorders)*, in *Magnesium in the Central Nervous System*, R. Vink and M. Nechifor, Editors. 2011, University of Adelaide Press

© 2011 The Authors.: Adelaide (AU).

427. *Nechifor M. Magnesium and Zinc in Bipolar Disorders. Biomed Pharmacol J 2023;16(1).*

428. Barbagallo, M., M. Belvedere, and L.J. Dominguez, *Magnesium homeostasis and aging.* Magnes Res, 2009. **22**(4): p. 235-46.

429. Kan, C., et al., *A systematic review and meta-analysis of the association between depression and insulin resistance.* Diabetes Care, 2013. **36**(2): p. 480-9.

430. Jeremiah, O.J., et al., *Evaluation of the effect of insulin sensitivity-enhancing lifestyle- and dietary-related adjuncts on antidepressant treatment response: protocol for a systematic review and meta-analysis.* Syst Rev, 2019. **8**(1): p. 62.

431. Tyagi, S., et al., *The peroxisome proliferator-activated receptor: A family of nuclear receptors role in various diseases.* J Adv Pharm Technol Res, 2011. **2**(4): p. 236-40.

432. Kang, S.W., et al., *Neuroprotective effects of magnesium-sulfate on ischemic injury mediated by modulating the release of glutamate and reduced of hyperreperfusion.* Brain Res, 2011. **1371**: p. 121-8.

433. Jamilian, M., et al., *Magnesium supplementation affects gene expression related to insulin and lipid in patients with gestational diabetes.* Magnes Res, 2017. **30**(3): p. 71-79.

434. Kumar, A.R. and P.A. Kurup, *Inhibition of membrane Na+-K+ ATPase activity: a common pathway in central nervous system disorders.* J Assoc Physicians India, 2002. **50**: p. 400-6.

435. Levine, J., et al., *High serum and cerebrospinal fluid Ca/Mg ratio in recently hospitalized acutely depressed patients.* Neuropsychobiology, 1999. **39**(2): p. 63-70.

436. Carman, J.S. and R.J. Wyatt, *Calcium: bivalent cation in the bivalent psychoses.* Biol Psychiatry, 1979. **14**(2): p. 295-336.

437. Banki, C.M., M. Arató, and C.D. Kilts, *Aminergic studies and cerebrospinal fluid cations in suicide.* Ann N Y Acad Sci, 1986. **487**: p. 221-30.

438. Gawryluk, J.W., et al., *Decreased levels of glutathione, the major brain antioxidant, in post-mortem prefrontal cortex from patients with psychiatric disorders.* Int J Neuropsychopharmacol, 2011. **14**(1): p. 123-30.

439. Sarandol, A., et al., *Major depressive disorder is accompanied with oxidative stress: short-term antidepressant treatment does not alter oxidative-antioxidative systems.* Hum Psychopharmacol, 2007. **22**(2): p. 67-73.

440. Belvederi Murri, M., et al., *The HPA axis in bipolar disorder: Systematic review and meta-analysis.* Psychoneuroendocrinology, 2016. **63**: p. 327-42.

441. Rybakowski, J.K. and K. Twardowska, *The dexamethasone/corticotropin-releasing hormone test in depression in bipolar and unipolar affective illness.* J Psychiatr Res, 1999. **33**(5): p. 363-70.

442. *U.S. Department of Health and Human Services. (n.d.-b). Schizophrenia. National Institute of Mental Health. https://www.nimh.nih.gov/health/statistics/schizophrenia.*

443. Kanofsky, J.D. and R. Sandyk, *Magnesium deficiency in chronic schizophrenia.* Int J Neurosci, 1991. **61**(1-2): p. 87-90.

444. *Seelig, M. S. (1986).Nutritional status and requirements of magnesium with considerations of individual differences and prevention of cardiovascular disease. Magnesium Bulletin, 8 , 171-185.*

445. Kirov, G.K. and K.N. Tsachev, *Magnesium, schizophrenia and manic-depressive disease.* Neuropsychobiology, 1990. **23**(2): p. 79-81.

446. Johnson, D., P. Blandina, and J. Goldfarb, *Glycine inhibition of glutamate evoked-release of norepinephrine in the hypothalamus is strychnine-insensitive.* Brain Res, 1994. **650**(1): p. 70-4.

447. McCutcheon, R.A., J.H. Krystal, and O.D. Howes, *Dopamine and glutamate in schizophrenia: biology, symptoms and treatment.* World Psychiatry, 2020. **19**(1): p. 15-33.

448. Maas, J.W., et al., *Studies of catecholamine metabolism in schizophrenia/psychosis--I.* Neuropsychopharmacology, 1993. **8**(2): p. 97-109.

449. *Centers for Disease Control and Prevention. (2023, September 27). What is ADHD?. Centers for Disease Control and Prevention. https://www.cdc.gov/ncbddd/adhd/facts.html.*

450. Hemamy, M., et al., *The effect of vitamin D and magnesium supplementation on the mental health status of attention-deficit hyperactive children: a randomized controlled trial.* BMC Pediatr, 2021. **21**(1): p. 178.

451. Effatpanah, M., et al., *Magnesium status and attention deficit hyperactivity disorder (ADHD): A meta-analysis.* Psychiatry Res, 2019. **274**: p. 228-234.

452. Kozielec, T. and B. Starobrat-Hermelin, *Assessment of magnesium levels in children with attention deficit hyperactivity disorder (ADHD).* Magnes Res, 1997. **10**(2): p. 143-8.

453. Cardoso, C.C., et al., *Evidence for the involvement of the monoaminergic system in the antidepressant-like effect of magnesium.* Prog Neuropsychopharmacol Biol Psychiatry, 2009. **33**(2): p. 235-42.

454. Gamo, N.J., M. Wang, and A.F. Arnsten, *Methylphenidate and atomoxetine enhance prefrontal function through α2-adrenergic and dopamine D1 receptors.* J Am Acad Child Adolesc Psychiatry, 2010. **49**(10): p. 1011-23.

455. *El Baza F, AlShahawi HA, Zahra S, AbdelHakim RA. Magnesium supplementation in children with attention deficit hyperactivity disorder. Egypt J Med Hum Genet. 2016;17:63–70.*

456. Mousain-Bosc, M., et al., *Magnesium VitB6 intake reduces central nervous system hyperexcitability in children.* J Am Coll Nutr, 2004. **23**(5): p. 545s-548s.

457. Starobrat-Hermelin, B. and T. Kozielec, *The effects of magnesium physiological supplementation on hyperactivity in children with attention deficit hyperactivity disorder (ADHD). Positive response to magnesium oral loading test.* Magnes Res, 1997. **10**(2): p. 149-56.

458. Sato, K., *Why is vitamin B6 effective in alleviating the symptoms of autism?* Med Hypotheses, 2018. **115**: p. 103-106.

459. Mousain-Bosc, M., et al., *Improvement of neurobehavioral disorders in children supplemented with magnesium-vitamin B6. I. Attention deficit hyperactivity disorders.* Magnes Res, 2006. **19**(1): p. 46-52.

460. Deng, X., et al., *Magnesium, vitamin D status and mortality: results from US National Health and Nutrition Examination Survey (NHANES) 2001 to 2006 and NHANES III.* BMC Med, 2013. **11**: p. 187.

461. Risco, F. and M.L. Traba, *Influence of magnesium on the in vitro synthesis of 24,25-dihydroxyvitamin D3 and 1 alpha, 25-dihydroxyvitamin D3.* Magnes Res, 1992. **5**(1): p. 5-14.

462. Hemamy, M., et al., *Effect of Vitamin D and Magnesium Supplementation on Behavior Problems in Children with Attention-Deficit Hyperactivity Disorder.* Int J Prev Med, 2020. **11**: p. 4.

463. *World Health Organization. (n.d.-c). Mental health: Neurological disorders. World Health Organization. https://www.who.int/news-room/questions-and-answers/item/mental-health-neurological-disorders#:~:text=These%20disorders%20include%20epilepsy%2C%20Alzheimer,trauma%2C%20and%20neurological%20disorders%20as.*

464. *GBD 2021 Nervous System Disorders Collaborators (2024). Global, regional, and national burden of disorders affecting the nervous system, 1990-2021: a systematic analysis for the Global Burden of Disease Study 2021. The Lancet. Neurology, 23(4), 344–381. https://doi.org/10.1016/S1474-4422(24)00038-3.*

465. Centers for Disease Control and Prevention. (2020, October 26). What is alzheimer's disease? Centers for Disease Control and Prevention. https://www.cdc.gov/aging/aginginfo/alzheimers.htm#:~:text=Alzheimer's%20disease%20is%20the%20most,thought%2C%20memory%2C%20and%20language.

466. Home: Alzheimer's association (no date) Alzheimer's Disease and Dementia. Available at: https://www.alz.org/ (Accessed: 27 April 2024).

467. Andrási, E., et al., Disturbances of magnesium concentrations in various brain areas in Alzheimer's disease. Magnes Res, 2000. 13(3): p. 189-96.

468. Du, K., et al., Association of Circulating Magnesium Levels in Patients With Alzheimer's Disease From 1991 to 2021: A Systematic Review and Meta-Analysis. Front Aging Neurosci, 2021. 13: p. 799824.

469. Alateeq, K., E.I. Walsh, and N. Cherbuin, Dietary magnesium intake is related to larger brain volumes and lower white matter lesions with notable sex differences. Eur J Nutr, 2023. 62(5): p. 2039-2051.

470. Yu, X., et al., By suppressing the expression of anterior pharynx-defective-1α and -1β and inhibiting the aggregation of β-amyloid protein, magnesium ions inhibit the cognitive decline of amyloid precursor protein/presenilin 1 transgenic mice. Faseb j, 2015. 29(12): p. 5044-58.

471. Nguyen, T.T., et al., Type 3 Diabetes and Its Role Implications in Alzheimer's Disease. Int J Mol Sci, 2020. 21(9).

472. Lee, H.J., et al., Diabetes and Alzheimer's Disease: Mechanisms and Nutritional Aspects. Clin Nutr Res, 2018. 7(4): p. 229-240.

473. Piuri, G., et al., Magnesium in Obesity, Metabolic Syndrome, and Type 2 Diabetes. Nutrients, 2021. 13(2).

474. Femminella, G.D., et al., Does insulin resistance influence neurodegeneration in non-diabetic Alzheimer's subjects? Alzheimers Res Ther, 2021. 13(1): p. 47.

475. Wang, P., et al., Magnesium ion influx reduces neuroinflammation in Aβ precursor protein/Presenilin 1 transgenic mice by suppressing the expression of interleukin-1β. Cell Mol Immunol, 2017. 14(5): p. 451-464.

476. Vassar, R., et al., The beta-secretase enzyme BACE in health and Alzheimer's disease: regulation, cell biology, function, and therapeutic potential. J Neurosci, 2009. 29(41): p. 12787-94.

477. Barbagallo, M., et al., Altered ionized magnesium levels in mild-to-moderate Alzheimer's disease. Magnes Res, 2011. 24(3): p. S115-21.

478. Vyklicky, V., et al., Structure, function, and pharmacology of NMDA receptor channels. Physiol Res, 2014. 63(Suppl 1): p. S191-203.

479. Xiong, Y., et al., Magnesium-L-threonate exhibited a neuroprotective effect against oxidative stress damage in HT22 cells and Alzheimer's disease mouse model. World J Psychiatry, 2022. 12(3): p. 410-424.

480. Ozturk, S. and A.E. Cillier, Magnesium supplementation in the treatment of dementia patients. Med Hypotheses, 2006. 67(5): p. 1223-5.

481. Ozawa, M., et al., Self-reported dietary intake of potassium, calcium, and magnesium and risk of dementia in the Japanese: the Hisayama Study. J Am Geriatr Soc, 2012. 60(8): p. 1515-20.

482. Parkinson's disease. AANS. (n.d.). https://www.aans.org/en/Patients/Neurosurgical-Conditions-and-Treatments/Parkinsons-Disease.

483. Bloem, B.R., M.S. Okun, and C. Klein, *Parkinson's disease.* Lancet, 2021. **397**(10291): p. 2284-2303.

484. Azman, K.F. and R. Zakaria, *Recent Advances on the Role of Brain-Derived Neurotrophic Factor (BDNF) in Neurodegenerative Diseases.* Int J Mol Sci, 2022. **23**(12).

485. Srinivasan, E., et al., *Alpha-Synuclein Aggregation in Parkinson's Disease.* Front Med (Lausanne), 2021. **8**: p. 736978.

486. Yasui, M., T. Kihira, and K. Ota, *Calcium, magnesium and aluminum concentrations in Parkinson's disease.* Neurotoxicology, 1992. **13**(3): p. 593-600.

487. Bocca, B., et al., *Metal changes in CSF and peripheral compartments of parkinsonian patients.* J Neurol Sci, 2006. **248**(1-2): p. 23-30.

488. Oyanagi, K., et al., *Magnesium deficiency over generations in rats with special references to the pathogenesis of the Parkinsonism-dementia complex and amyotrophic lateral sclerosis of Guam.* Neuropathology, 2006. **26**(2): p. 115-28.

489. Raj, K., et al., *Metals associated neurodegeneration in Parkinson's disease: Insight to physiological, pathological mechanisms and management.* Neurosci Lett, 2021. **753**: p. 135873.

490. Lingam, I. and N.J. Robertson, *Magnesium as a Neuroprotective Agent: A Review of Its Use in the Fetus, Term Infant with Neonatal Encephalopathy, and the Adult Stroke Patient.* Dev Neurosci, 2018. **40**(1): p. 1-12.

491. Zhao, Y., et al., *Metal Exposure and Risk of Parkinson Disease: A Systematic Review and Meta-Analysis.* Am J Epidemiol, 2023. **192**(7): p. 1207-1223.

492. Kozielec, T., A. Sałacka, and B. Karakiewicz, *The influence of magnesium supplementation on concentrations of chosen bioelements and toxic metals in adult human hair. Magnesium and chosen bioelements in hair.* Magnes Res, 2004. **17**(3): p. 183-8.

493. Shen, Y., et al., *Treatment Of Magnesium-L-Threonate Elevates The Magnesium Level In The Cerebrospinal Fluid And Attenuates Motor Deficits And Dopamine Neuron Loss In A Mouse Model Of Parkinson's disease.* Neuropsychiatr Dis Treat, 2019. **15**: p. 3143-3153.

494. *Sian J, Youdim MBH, Riederer P, et al. MPTP-Induced Parkinsonian Syndrome. In: Siegel GJ, Agranoff BW, Albers RW, et al., editors. Basic Neurochemistry: Molecular, Cellular and Medical Aspects. 6th edition. Philadelphia: Lippincott-Raven; 1999. Available from: https://www.ncbi.nlm.nih.gov/books/NBK27974/.*

495. *U.S. Department of Health and Human Services. (n.d.). Amyotrophic lateral sclerosis (ALS). National Institute of Neurological Disorders and Stroke. https://www.ninds.nih.gov/health-information/disorders/amyotrophic-lateral-sclerosis-als.*

496. Hermosura, M.C., et al., *A TRPM7 variant shows altered sensitivity to magnesium that may contribute to the pathogenesis of two Guamanian neurodegenerative disorders.* Proc Natl Acad Sci U S A, 2005. **102**(32): p. 11510-5.

497. Yasui, M., et al., *Aluminum deposition in the central nervous system of patients with amyotrophic lateral sclerosis from the Kii Peninsula of Japan.* Neurotoxicology, 1991. **12**(3): p. 615-20.

498. *Centers for Disease Control and Prevention. (2023a, September 7). Traumatic brain injury / concussion. Centers for Disease Control and Prevention. https://www.cdc.gov/traumaticbraininjury/index.html.*

499. Sen, A.P. and A. Gulati, *Use of magnesium in traumatic brain injury.* Neurotherapeutics, 2010. **7**(1): p. 91-9.

500. *Turner, Renee & Vink, Robert. (2012). Magnesium and Traumatic Brain Injury.* 10.1007/978-1-62703-044-1_18.

501. *Institute of Medicine (US) Committee on Nutrition, Trauma, and the Brain; Erdman J, Oria M, Pillsbury L, editors. Nutrition and Traumatic Brain Injury: Improving Acute and Subacute Health Outcomes in Military Personnel. Washington (DC): National Academies Press (US); 2011. 12, Magnesium. Available from: https://www.ncbi.nlm.nih.gov/books/NBK209305/.*

502. Fromm, L., et al., *Magnesium attenuates post-traumatic depression/anxiety following diffuse traumatic brain injury in rats.* J Am Coll Nutr, 2004. **23**(5): p. 529s-533s.

503. Arango, M.F. and D. Bainbridge, *Magnesium for acute traumatic brain injury.* Cochrane Database Syst Rev, 2008(4): p. Cd005400.

504. *DhandapaniSS, GuptaA, VivekanandhanS, SharmaBS, MahapatraAK. Randomized controlled trial of magnesium sulphate in severe closed traumatic brain injury. Indian J Neurotrauma 5: 27–33, 2008.*

505. *Jain S, Iverson LM. Glasgow Coma Scale. [Updated 2023 Jun 12]. In: StatPearls [Internet]. Treasure Island (FL): StatPearls Publishing; 2024 Jan-. Available from: https://www.ncbi.nlm.nih.gov/books/NBK513298/.*

506. Shogi, T., et al., *Effects of a low extracellular magnesium concentration and endotoxin on IL-1beta and TNF-alpha release from, and mRNA levels in, isolated rat alveolar macrophages.* Magnes Res, 2002. **15**(3-4): p. 147-52.

507. Hutchinson, P.J., et al., *Inflammation in human brain injury: intracerebral concentrations of IL-1alpha, IL-1beta, and their endogenous inhibitor IL-1ra.* J Neurotrauma, 2007. **24**(10): p. 1545-57.

508. Morganti-Kossman, M.C., et al., *Production of cytokines following brain injury: beneficial and deleterious for the damaged tissue.* Mol Psychiatry, 1997. **2**(2): p. 133-6.

509. Filippi, M., et al., *Multiple sclerosis.* Nat Rev Dis Primers, 2018. **4**(1): p. 43.

510. *U.S. Department of Health and Human Services. (n.d.-b). Multiple sclerosis. National Institute of Neurological Disorders and Stroke. https://www.ninds.nih.gov/health-information/disorders/multiple-sclerosis.*

511. Yasui, M. and K. Ota, *Experimental and clinical studies on dysregulation of magnesium metabolism and the aetiopathogenesis of multiple sclerosis.* Magnes Res, 1992. **5**(4): p. 295-302.

512. Reddy, P. and L.R. Edwards, *Magnesium Supplementation in Vitamin D Deficiency.* Am J Ther, 2019. **26**(1): p. e124-e132.

513. Cheung, M.M., et al., *The effect of combined magnesium and vitamin D supplementation on vitamin D status, systemic inflammation, and blood pressure: A randomized double-blinded controlled trial.* Nutrition, 2022. **99-100**: p. 111674.

514. Goldberg, P., M.C. Fleming, and E.H. Picard, *Multiple sclerosis: decreased relapse rate through dietary supplementation with calcium, magnesium and vitamin D.* Med Hypotheses, 1986. **21**(2): p. 193-200.

515. *Epilepsy. AANS. (n.d.). https://www.aans.org/en/Patients/Neurosurgical-Conditions-and-Treatments/Epilepsy.*

516. Barker-Haliski, M. and H.S. White, *Glutamatergic Mechanisms Associated with Seizures and Epilepsy.* Cold Spring Harb Perspect Med, 2015. **5**(8): p. a022863.

517. Chen, B.B., et al., *Seizures Related to Hypomagnesemia: A Case Series and Review of the Literature.* Child Neurol Open, 2016. **3**: p. 2329048x16674834.

518. Yuen, A.W. and J.W. Sander, *Can magnesium supplementation reduce seizures in people with epilepsy? A hypothesis.* Epilepsy Res, 2012. **100**(1-2): p. 152-6.

519. Osborn, K.E., et al., *Addressing potential role of magnesium dyshomeostasis to improve treatment efficacy for epilepsy: A reexamination of the literature.* J Clin Pharmacol, 2016. **56**(3): p. 260-5.

520. Saghazadeh, A., et al., *Possible role of trace elements in epilepsy and febrile seizures: a meta-analysis.* Nutr Rev, 2015. **73**(11): p. 760-79.

521. Gupta, S.K., et al., *Serum magnesium levels in idiopathic epilepsy.* J Assoc Physicians India, 1994. **42**(6): p. 456-7.

522. Zou, L.P., et al., *Three-week combination treatment with ACTH + magnesium sulfate versus ACTH monotherapy for infantile spasms: a 24-week, randomized, open-label, follow-up study in China.* Clin Ther, 2010. **32**(4): p. 692-700.

523. Boulis, M., M. Boulis, and D. Clauw, *Magnesium and Fibromyalgia: A Literature Review.* J Prim Care Community Health, 2021. **12**: p. 21501327211038433.

524. Bagis, S., et al., *Is magnesium citrate treatment effective on pain, clinical parameters and functional status in patients with fibromyalgia?* Rheumatol Int, 2013. **33**(1): p. 167-72.

525. Littlejohn, G. and E. Guymer, *Modulation of NMDA Receptor Activity in Fibromyalgia.* Biomedicines, 2017. **5**(2).

526. Engen, D.J., et al., *Effects of transdermal magnesium chloride on quality of life for patients with fibromyalgia: a feasibility study.* J Integr Med, 2015. **13**(5): p. 306-13.

527. *U.S. Department of Health and Human Services. (n.d.-b). Migraine. National Institute of Neurological Disorders and Stroke. https://www.ninds.nih.gov/health-information/disorders/migraine.*

528. Domitrz, I. and J. Cegielska, *Magnesium as an Important Factor in the Pathogenesis and Treatment of Migraine-From Theory to Practice.* Nutrients, 2022. **14**(5).

529. Goadsby, P.J., et al., *Pathophysiology of Migraine: A Disorder of Sensory Processing.* Physiol Rev, 2017. **97**(2): p. 553-622.

530. Hoffmann, J. and A. Charles, *Glutamate and Its Receptors as Therapeutic Targets for Migraine.* Neurotherapeutics, 2018. **15**(2): p. 361-370.

531. Welch, K.M. and N.M. Ramadan, *Mitochondria, magnesium and migraine.* J Neurol Sci, 1995. **134**(1-2): p. 9-14.

532. Trauninger, A., et al., *Oral magnesium load test in patients with migraine.* Headache, 2002. **42**(2): p. 114-9.

533. Chiu, H.Y., et al., *Effects of Intravenous and Oral Magnesium on Reducing Migraine: A Meta-analysis of Randomized Controlled Trials.* Pain Physician, 2016. **19**(1): p. E97-112.

534. Mauskop, A., et al., *Deficiency in serum ionized magnesium but not total magnesium in patients with migraines. Possible role of ICa2+/IMg2+ ratio.* Headache, 1993. **33**(3): p. 135-8.

535. Antonaci, F., et al., *A review of current European treatment guidelines for migraine.* J Headache Pain, 2010. **11**(1): p. 13-9.

536. *Menstrual migraine treatment and prevention: AMF. American Migraine Foundation. (2022, November 29). https://americanmigrainefoundation.org/resource-library/menstrual-migraine-treatment-and-prevention/.*

537. Facchinetti, F., et al., *Magnesium prophylaxis of menstrual migraine: effects on intracellular magnesium.* Headache, 1991. **31**(5): p. 298-301.

538. Wang, Z., et al., *Metabolic disorders and risk of cardiovascular diseases: a two-sample mendelian randomization study.* BMC Cardiovasc Disord, 2023. **23**(1): p. 529.

539. Phillips, M.C., *Metabolic Strategies in Healthcare: A New Era.* Aging Dis, 2022. **13**(3): p. 655-672.

540. *Facts & figures (2024) International Diabetes Federation. Available at: https://idf.org/about-diabetes/diabetes-facts-figures/ (Accessed: 26 May 2024).*

541. Barbagallo, M. and L.J. Dominguez, *Magnesium and type 2 diabetes.* World J Diabetes, 2015. **6**(10): p. 1152-7.

542. Lee, S.H., S.Y. Park, and C.S. Choi, *Insulin Resistance: From Mechanisms to Therapeutic Strategies.* Diabetes Metab J, 2022. **46**(1): p. 15-37.

543. *Freeman AM, Acevedo LA, Pennings N. Insulin Resistance. [Updated 2023 Aug 17]. In: StatPearls [Internet]. Treasure Island (FL): StatPearls Publishing; 2024 Jan-. Available from: https://www.ncbi.nlm.nih.gov/books/NBK507839/#.*

544. Kostov, K., *Effects of Magnesium Deficiency on Mechanisms of Insulin Resistance in Type 2 Diabetes: Focusing on the Processes of Insulin Secretion and Signaling.* Int J Mol Sci, 2019. **20**(6).

545. Ishizuka, J., et al., *In vitro relationship between magnesium and insulin secretion.* Magnes Res, 1994. **7**(1): p. 17-22.

546. Gopinath, P., V. Ramalingam, and R. Breslow, *Magnesium pyrophosphates in enzyme mimics of nucleotide synthases and kinases and in their prebiotic chemistry.* Proc Natl Acad Sci U S A, 2015. **112**(39): p. 12011-4.

547. Toto, K.H. and C.B. Yucha, *Magnesium: homeostasis, imbalances, and therapeutic uses.* Crit Care Nurs Clin North Am, 1994. **6**(4): p. 767-83.

548. Rosolová, H., O. Mayer, Jr., and G.M. Reaven, *Insulin-mediated glucose disposal is decreased in normal subjects with relatively low plasma magnesium concentrations.* Metabolism, 2000. **49**(3): p. 418-20.

549. Takaya, J., H. Higashino, and Y. Kobayashi, *Intracellular magnesium and insulin resistance.* Magnes Res, 2004. **17**(2): p. 126-36.

550. Chutia, H. and K.G. Lynrah, *Association of Serum Magnesium Deficiency with Insulin Resistance in Type 2 Diabetes Mellitus.* J Lab Physicians, 2015. **7**(2): p. 75-8.

551. Lefébvre, P.J., G. Paolisso, and A.J. Scheen, *[Magnesium and glucose metabolism].* Therapie, 1994. **49**(1): p. 1-7.

552. Swaminathan, R., *Magnesium metabolism and its disorders.* Clin Biochem Rev, 2003. **24**(2): p. 47-66.

553. Chen, L., et al., *Mechanisms Linking Inflammation to Insulin Resistance.* Int J Endocrinol, 2015. **2015**: p. 508409.

554. *Voma C., Romani A.M. Role of Magnesium in the Regulation of Hepatic Glucose Homeostasis. InTech; London, UK: 2014. pp. 95–111.*

555. Morais, J.B.S., et al., *Effect of magnesium supplementation on insulin resistance in humans: A systematic review.* Nutrition, 2017. **38**: p. 54-60.

556. Simental-Mendía, L.E., et al., *A systematic review and meta-analysis of randomized controlled trials on the effects of magnesium supplementation on insulin sensitivity and glucose control.* Pharmacol Res, 2016. **111**: p. 272-282.

557. Cahill, F., et al., *High dietary magnesium intake is associated with low insulin resistance in the Newfoundland population.* PLoS One, 2013. **8**(3): p. e58278.

558. Djurhuus, M.S., et al., *Insulin increases renal magnesium excretion: a possible cause of magnesium depletion in hyperinsulinaemic states.* Diabet Med, 1995. **12**(8): p. 664-9.

559. van Gerwen, J., A.S. Shun-Shion, and D.J. Fazakerley, *Insulin signalling and GLUT4 trafficking in insulin resistance.* Biochem Soc Trans, 2023. **51**(3): p. 1057-1069.

560. Govers, R., *Molecular mechanisms of GLUT4 regulation in adipocytes.* Diabetes Metab, 2014. **40**(6): p. 400-10.

561. Oost, L.J., et al., *Magnesium increases insulin-dependent glucose uptake in adipocytes.* Front Endocrinol (Lausanne), 2022. **13**: p. 986616.

562. Fahed, G., et al., *Metabolic Syndrome: Updates on Pathophysiology and Management in 2021.* Int J Mol Sci, 2022. **23**(2).

563. Reaven, G.M., *Banting lecture 1988. Role of insulin resistance in human disease.* Diabetes, 1988. **37**(12): p. 1595-607.

564. *What is metabolic syndrome? (no date) National Heart Lung and Blood Institute. Available at: https://www.nhlbi.nih.gov/health/metabolic-syndrome#:~:text=Metabolic%20syndrome%20is%20common%20in,health%20problems%20it%20can%20cause. (Accessed: 03 June 2024).*

565. Corica, F., et al., *Serum ionized magnesium levels in relation to metabolic syndrome in type 2 diabetic patients.* J Am Coll Nutr, 2006. **25**(3): p. 210-5.

566. Guerrero-Romero, F. and M. Rodríguez-Morán, *Hypomagnesemia, oxidative stress, inflammation, and metabolic syndrome.* Diabetes Metab Res Rev, 2006. **22**(6): p. 471-6.

567. Guerrero-Romero, F. and M. Rodríguez-Morán, *Low serum magnesium levels and metabolic syndrome.* Acta Diabetol, 2002. **39**(4): p. 209-13.

568. La, S.A., et al., *Low Magnesium Levels in Adults with Metabolic Syndrome: a Meta-Analysis.* Biol Trace Elem Res, 2016. **170**(1): p. 33-42.

569. Pelczyńska, M., M. Moszak, and P. Bogdański, *The Role of Magnesium in the Pathogenesis of Metabolic Disorders.* Nutrients, 2022. **14**(9).

570. *Obesity and Overweight. Available online: https://www.who.int/news-room/fact-sheets/detail/obesity-and-overweight (accessed May 26, 2024).*

571. Lefebvre, P., et al., *Nutrient deficiencies in patients with obesity considering bariatric surgery: a cross-sectional study.* Surg Obes Relat Dis, 2014. **10**(3): p. 540-6.

572. Babapour, M., et al., *Associations Between Serum Magnesium Concentrations and Polycystic Ovary Syndrome Status: a Systematic Review and Meta-analysis.* Biol Trace Elem Res, 2021. **199**(4): p. 1297-1305.

573. *Shamnani, G.; Rukadikar, C.; Gupta, V.; Singh, S.; Tiwari, S.; Bhartiy, S.; Sharma, P. Serum Magnesium in Relation with Obesity. Natl. J. Physiol. Pharm. Pharmacol. 2018, 8, 1074–1077.*

574. Hassan, S.A.U., et al., *Comparison of Serum Magnesium Levels in Overweight and Obese Children and Normal Weight Children.* Cureus, 2017. **9**(8): p. e1607.

575. Peuhkuri, K., H. Vapaatalo, and R. Korpela, *Even low-grade inflammation impacts on small intestinal function.* World J Gastroenterol, 2010. **16**(9): p. 1057-62.

576. Dibaba, D.T., et al., *Dietary magnesium intake and risk of metabolic syndrome: a meta-analysis.* Diabet Med, 2014. **31**(11): p. 1301-9.

577. Farhanghi, M.A., S. Mahboob, and A. Ostadrahimi, *Obesity induced magnesium deficiency can be treated by vitamin D supplementation.* J Pak Med Assoc, 2009. **59**(4): p. 258-61.

578. Rayssiguier, Y., et al., *High fructose consumption combined with low dietary magnesium intake may increase the incidence of the metabolic syndrome by inducing inflammation.* Magnes Res, 2006. **19**(4): p. 237-43.

579. Lu, L., et al., *Magnesium intake is inversely associated with risk of obesity in a 30-year prospective follow-up study among American young adults.* Eur J Nutr, 2020. **59**(8): p. 3745-3753.

580. Guerrero-Romero, F., C. Bermudez-Peña, and M. Rodríguez-Morán, *Severe hypomagnesemia and low-grade inflammation in metabolic syndrome.* Magnes Res, 2011. **24**(2): p. 45-53.

581. Ellulu, M.S., et al., *Obesity and inflammation: the linking mechanism and the complications.* Arch Med Sci, 2017. **13**(4): p. 851-863.

582. Dai, Q., et al., *Magnesium status and supplementation influence vitamin D status and metabolism: results from a randomized trial.* Am J Clin Nutr, 2018. **108**(6): p. 1249-1258.

583. Stokic, E., et al., *Chronic Latent Magnesium Deficiency in Obesity Decreases Positive Effects of Vitamin D on Cardiometabolic Risk Indicators.* Curr Vasc Pharmacol, 2018. **16**(6): p. 610-617.

584. *Hypertension. Available online: https://www.who.int/news-room/fact-sheets/detail/hypertension.*

585. Han, H., et al., *Dose-response relationship between dietary magnesium intake, serum magnesium concentration and risk of hypertension: a systematic review and meta-analysis of prospective cohort studies.* Nutr J, 2017. **16**(1): p. 26.

586. Rayssiguier, Y., et al., *Magnesium deficiency and metabolic syndrome: stress and inflammation may reflect calcium activation.* Magnes Res, 2010. **23**(2): p. 73-80.

587. Zhou, M.S., A. Wang, and H. Yu, *Link between insulin resistance and hypertension: What is the evidence from evolutionary biology?* Diabetol Metab Syndr, 2014. **6**(1): p. 12.

588. Asbaghi, O., et al., *The Effects of Magnesium Supplementation on Blood Pressure and Obesity Measure Among Type 2 Diabetes Patient: a Systematic Review and Meta-analysis of Randomized Controlled Trials.* Biol Trace Elem Res, 2021. **199**(2): p. 413-424.

589. Dibaba, D.T., et al., *The effect of magnesium supplementation on blood pressure in individuals with insulin resistance, prediabetes, or noncommunicable chronic diseases: a meta-analysis of randomized controlled trials.* Am J Clin Nutr, 2017. **106**(3): p. 921-929.

590. Bitzur, R., et al., *Triglycerides and HDL cholesterol: stars or second leads in diabetes?* Diabetes Care, 2009. **32 Suppl 2**(Suppl 2): p. S373-7.

591. Itoh, K., T. Kawasaka, and M. Nakamura, *The effects of high oral magnesium supplementation on blood pressure, serum lipids and related variables in apparently healthy Japanese subjects.* Br J Nutr, 1997. **78**(5): p. 737-50.

592. Rayssiguier, Y., et al., *Effect of magnesium deficiency on post-heparin lipase activity and tissue lipoprotein lipase in the rat.* Lipids, 1991. **26**(3): p. 182-6.

593. Salehidoost, R., et al., *Effect of oral magnesium supplement on cardiometabolic markers in people with prediabetes: a double blind randomized controlled clinical trial.* Sci Rep, 2022. **12**(1): p. 18209.

594. Elin, R.J., *Assessment of magnesium status for diagnosis and therapy.* Magnes Res, 2010. **23**(4): p. S194-8.

595. Guerrero-Romero, F., et al., *Oral magnesium supplementation improves insulin sensitivity in non-diabetic subjects with insulin resistance. A double-blind placebo-controlled randomized trial.* Diabetes Metab, 2004. **30**(3): p. 253-8.

596. Veronese, N., et al., *Effect of magnesium supplementation on glucose metabolism in people with or at risk of diabetes: a systematic review and meta-analysis of double-blind randomized controlled trials.* Eur J Clin Nutr, 2016. **70**(12): p. 1354-1359.

597. *Diabetes (no date) World Health Organization. Available at: https://www.who.int/news-room/fact-sheets/detail/diabetes (Accessed: 10 June 2024).*

598. Modzelewski, R., et al., *Gestational Diabetes Mellitus-Recent Literature Review.* J Clin Med, 2022. **11**(19).

599. Krause, M. and G. De Vito, *Type 1 and Type 2 Diabetes Mellitus: Commonalities, Differences and the Importance of Exercise and Nutrition.* Nutrients, 2023. **15**(19).

600. Dong, J.Y., et al., *Magnesium intake and risk of type 2 diabetes: meta-analysis of prospective cohort studies.* Diabetes Care, 2011. **34**(9): p. 2116-22.

601. Bertinato, J., K.C. Wang, and S. Hayward, *Serum Magnesium Concentrations in the Canadian Population and Associations with Diabetes, Glycemic Regulation, and Insulin Resistance.* Nutrients, 2017. **9**(3).

602. Barbagallo, M. and L.J. Dominguez, *Magnesium metabolism in type 2 diabetes mellitus, metabolic syndrome and insulin resistance.* Arch Biochem Biophys, 2007. **458**(1): p. 40-7.

603. Paolisso, G., et al., *Magnesium and glucose homeostasis.* Diabetologia, 1990. **33**(9): p. 511-4.

604. Esmeralda, C.A.C., et al., *Deranged Fractional Excretion of Magnesium and Serum Magnesium Levels in Relation to Retrograde Glycaemic Regulation in Patients with Type 2 Diabetes Mellitus.* Curr Diabetes Rev, 2021. **17**(1): p. 91-100.

605. Dasgupta, A., D. Sarma, and U.K. Saikia, *Hypomagnesemia in type 2 diabetes mellitus.* Indian J Endocrinol Metab, 2012. **16**(6): p. 1000-3.

606. Hruby, A., et al., *Magnesium Intake, Quality of Carbohydrates, and Risk of Type 2 Diabetes: Results From Three U.S. Cohorts.* Diabetes Care, 2017. **40**(12): p. 1695-1702.

607. Nicholson, K.M. and N.G. Anderson, *The protein kinase B/Akt signalling pathway in human malignancy.* Cell Signal, 2002. **14**(5): p. 381-95.

608. Gommers, L.M., et al., *Hypomagnesemia in Type 2 Diabetes: A Vicious Circle?* Diabetes, 2016. **65**(1): p. 3-13.

609. Feng, J., et al., *Role of Magnesium in Type 2 Diabetes Mellitus.* Biol Trace Elem Res, 2020. **196**(1): p. 74-85.

610. Bherwani, S., et al., *Hypomagnesaemia: a modifiable risk factor of diabetic nephropathy.* Horm Mol Biol Clin Investig, 2017. **29**(3): p. 79-84.

611. Prabodh, S., et al., *Status of copper and magnesium levels in diabetic nephropathy cases: a case-control study from South India.* Biol Trace Elem Res, 2011. **142**(1): p. 29-35.

612. Pham, P.C., et al., *Lower serum magnesium levels are associated with more rapid decline of renal function in patients with diabetes mellitus type 2.* Clin Nephrol, 2005. **63**(6): p. 429-36.

613. Pop-Busui, R., et al., *Impact of glycemic control strategies on the progression of diabetic peripheral neuropathy in the Bypass Angioplasty Revascularization Investigation 2 Diabetes (BARI 2D) Cohort.* Diabetes Care, 2013. **36**(10): p. 3208-15.

614. Boulton, A.J., et al., *The global burden of diabetic foot disease.* Lancet, 2005. **366**(9498): p. 1719-24.

615. Keşkek, S.O., et al., *Low serum magnesium levels and diabetic foot ulcers.* Pak J Med Sci, 2013. **29**(6): p. 1329-33.

616. Razzaghi, R., et al., *Magnesium Supplementation and the Effects on Wound Healing and Metabolic Status in Patients with Diabetic Foot Ulcer: a Randomized, Double-Blind, Placebo-Controlled Trial.* Biol Trace Elem Res, 2018. **181**(2): p. 207-215.

617. Villegas, R., et al., *Dietary calcium and magnesium intakes and the risk of type 2 diabetes: the Shanghai Women's Health Study.* Am J Clin Nutr, 2009. **89**(4): p. 1059-67.

618. Agrawal, P., et al., *Association of macrovascular complications of type 2 diabetes mellitus with serum magnesium levels.* Diabetes Metab Syndr, 2011. **5**(1): p. 41-4.

619. Wang, S., et al., *Serum electrolyte levels in relation to macrovascular complications in Chinese patients with diabetes mellitus.* Cardiovasc Diabetol, 2013. **12**: p. 146.

620. Hata, A., et al., *Magnesium intake decreases Type 2 diabetes risk through the improvement of insulin resistance and inflammation: the Hisayama Study.* Diabet Med, 2013. **30**(12): p. 1487-94.

621. Sohrabipour, S., et al., *Effect of magnesium sulfate administration to improve insulin resistance in type 2 diabetes animal model: using the hyperinsulinemic-euglycemic clamp technique.* Fundam Clin Pharmacol, 2018. **32**(6): p. 603-616.

622. Kumawat, M., et al., *Antioxidant Enzymes and Lipid Peroxidation in Type 2 Diabetes Mellitus Patients with and without Nephropathy.* N Am J Med Sci, 2013. **5**(3): p. 213-9.

623. Yang, H., et al., *Oxidative stress and diabetes mellitus.* Clin Chem Lab Med, 2011. **49**(11): p. 1773-82.

624. Liu, M., et al., *Magnesium supplementation improves diabetic mitochondrial and cardiac diastolic function.* JCI Insight, 2019. **4**(1).

625. Saad, M.J., A. Santos, and P.O. Prada, *Linking Gut Microbiota and Inflammation to Obesity and Insulin Resistance.* Physiology (Bethesda), 2016. **31**(4): p. 283-93.

626. Caesar, R., *Pharmacologic and Nonpharmacologic Therapies for the Gut Microbiota in Type 2 Diabetes.* Can J Diabetes, 2019. **43**(3): p. 224-231.

627. Thingholm, L.B., et al., *Obese Individuals with and without Type 2 Diabetes Show Different Gut Microbial Functional Capacity and Composition.* Cell Host Microbe, 2019. **26**(2): p. 252-264.e10.

628. Jovanovic-Peterson, L. and C.M. Peterson, *Vitamin and mineral deficiencies which may predispose to glucose intolerance of pregnancy.* J Am Coll Nutr, 1996. **15**(1): p. 14-20.

629. Luo, L., et al., *The efficacy of magnesium supplementation for gestational diabetes: A meta-analysis of randomized controlled trials.* Eur J Obstet Gynecol Reprod Biol, 2024. **293**: p. 84-90.

630. Qu, Q., R. Rong, and J. Yu, *Effect of magnesium supplementation on pregnancy outcome in gestational diabetes mellitus patients: A meta-analysis of randomized controlled trials.* Food Sci Nutr, 2022. **10**(10): p. 3193-3202.

631. Song, Y., et al., *Effects of oral magnesium supplementation on glycaemic control in Type 2 diabetes: a meta-analysis of randomized double-blind controlled trials.* Diabet Med, 2006. **23**(10): p. 1050-6.

632. Guerrero-Romero, F. and M. Rodríguez-Morán, *[Oral magnesium supplementation: an adjuvant alternative to facing the worldwide challenge of type 2 diabetes?].* Cir Cir, 2014. **82**(3): p. 282-9.

633. Zghoul, N., et al., *Hypomagnesemia in diabetes patients: comparison of serum and intracellular measurement of responses to magnesium supplementation and its role in inflammation.* Diabetes Metab Syndr Obes, 2018. **11**: p. 389-400.

634. Fang, X., et al., *Dose-Response Relationship between Dietary Magnesium Intake and Risk of Type 2 Diabetes Mellitus: A Systematic Review and Meta-Regression Analysis of Prospective Cohort Studies.* Nutrients, 2016. **8**(11).

635. *Bone Health and osteoporosis: What it means to you (2023) National Institute of Arthritis and Musculoskeletal and Skin Diseases. Available at: https://www.niams.nih.gov/health-topics/surgeon-generals-report-bone-health-and-osteoporosis-what-it-means-you (Accessed: 01 July 2024).*

636. *Signs and symptoms: Osteoporosis canada (2022) Osteoporosis Canada |. Available at: https://osteoporosis.ca/signs-and-symptoms/ (Accessed: 01 July 2024).*

637. *Bone diseases (no date) MedlinePlus. Available at: https://medlineplus.gov/bonediseases.html#:~:text=Different%20kinds%20of%20bone%20prob lems,of%20bone%20makes%20them%20weak (Accessed: 01 July 2024).*

638. Castiglioni, S., et al., *Magnesium and osteoporosis: current state of knowledge and future research directions.* Nutrients, 2013. **5**(8): p. 3022-33.

639. *Medical News Today. (2023). Hydroxyapatite: What is it and how can it affect your bones? Medical News Today. Retrieved June 26, 2024, from https://www.medicalnewstoday.com/articles/hydroxyapatite-bone.*

640. Surowiec, R.K., M.R. Allen, and J.M. Wallace, *Bone hydration: How we can evaluate it, what can it tell us, and is it an effective therapeutic target?* Bone Rep, 2022. **16**: p. 101161.

641. Al Alawi, A.M., S.W. Majoni, and H. Falhammar, *Magnesium and Human Health: Perspectives and Research Directions.* Int J Endocrinol, 2018. **2018**: p. 9041694.

642. Rachner, T.D., S. Khosla, and L.C. Hofbauer, *Osteoporosis: now and the future.* Lancet, 2011. **377**(9773): p. 1276-87.

643. *Bone Mineral Density Testing: Osteoporosis Canada (2021) Osteoporosis Canada |. Available at: https://osteoporosis.ca/bone-mineral-density-testing/ (Accessed: 12 July 2024).*

644. Karlamangla, A.S., S.M. Burnett-Bowie, and C.J. Crandall, *Bone Health During the Menopause Transition and Beyond.* Obstet Gynecol Clin North Am, 2018. **45**(4): p. 695-708.

645. Nieves, J.W., *Osteoporosis: the role of micronutrients.* Am J Clin Nutr, 2005. **81**(5): p. 1232s-1239s.

646. Uwitonze, A.M. and M.S. Razzaque, *Role of Magnesium in Vitamin D Activation and Function.* J Am Osteopath Assoc, 2018. **118**(3): p. 181-189.

647. *Wikipedia contributors. (n.d.). Trabecula. In Wikipedia, The Free Encyclopedia. Retrieved June 29, 2024, from https://en.wikipedia.org/wiki/Trabecula#:~:text=Bone%20trabecula-,Structure,and%20plates%20of%20bone%20tissue.*

648. Sadat-Ali, M., et al., *Tibial cortical thickness: A dependable tool for assessing osteoporosis in the absence of dual energy X-ray absorptiometry.* Int J Appl Basic Med Res, 2015. **5**(1): p. 21-4.

649. Steidl, L., R. Ditmar, and R. Kubícek, *[Biochemical findings in osteoporosis. I. The significance of magnesium].* Cas Lek Cesk, 1990. **129**(2): p. 51-5.

650. Ishii, A. and Y. Imanishi, *[Magnesium disorder in metabolic bone diseases].* Clin Calcium, 2012. **22**(8): p. 1251-6.

651. Belluci, M.M., et al., *Magnesium deficiency results in an increased formation of osteoclasts.* J Nutr Biochem, 2013. **24**(8): p. 1488-98.

652. Mori, S., et al., *Hypomagnesemia with increased metabolism of parathyroid hormone and reduced responsiveness to calcitropic hormones.* Intern Med, 1992. **31**(6): p. 820-4.

653. Baker-LePain, J.C., M.C. Nakamura, and N.E. Lane, *Effects of inflammation on bone: an update.* Curr Opin Rheumatol, 2011. **23**(4): p. 389-95.

654. Li, F.X., et al., *The Role of Substance P in the Regulation of Bone and Cartilage Metabolic Activity.* Front Endocrinol (Lausanne), 2020. **11**: p. 77.

655. Orchard, T.S., et al., *Magnesium intake, bone mineral density, and fractures: results from the Women's Health Initiative Observational Study.* Am J Clin Nutr, 2014. **99**(4): p. 926-33.

656. Chang, J., et al., *The Association Between the Concentration of Serum Magnesium and Postmenopausal Osteoporosis.* Front Med (Lausanne), 2020. **7**: p. 381.

657. Erem, S., A. Atfi, and M.S. Razzaque, *Anabolic effects of vitamin D and magnesium in aging bone.* J Steroid Biochem Mol Biol, 2019. **193**: p. 105400.

658. Rosanoff, A., Q. Dai, and S.A. Shapses, *Essential Nutrient Interactions: Does Low or Suboptimal Magnesium Status Interact with Vitamin D and/or Calcium Status?* Adv Nutr, 2016. **7**(1): p. 25-43.

659. Lips, P., *Vitamin D deficiency and secondary hyperparathyroidism in the elderly: consequences for bone loss and fractures and therapeutic implications.* Endocr Rev, 2001. **22**(4): p. 477-501.

660. Muñoz-Garach, A., B. García-Fontana, and M. Muñoz-Torres, *Nutrients and Dietary Patterns Related to Osteoporosis.* Nutrients, 2020. **12**(7).

661. Ditmar, R. and L. Steidl, *[The significance of magnesium in orthopedics. V. Magnesium in osteoporosis].* Acta Chir Orthop Traumatol Cech, 1989. **56**(2): p. 143-59.

662. Wallach, S., *Effects of magnesium on skeletal metabolism.* Magnes Trace Elem, 1990. **9**(1): p. 1-14.

663. Fatemi, S., et al., *Effect of experimental human magnesium depletion on parathyroid hormone secretion and 1,25-dihydroxyvitamin D metabolism.* J Clin Endocrinol Metab, 1991. **73**(5): p. 1067-72.

664. Rude, R.K., et al., *Dietary magnesium reduction to 25% of nutrient requirement disrupts bone and mineral metabolism in the rat.* Bone, 2005. **37**(2): p. 211-9.

665. Rude, R.K., et al., *Reduction of dietary magnesium by only 50% in the rat disrupts bone and mineral metabolism.* Osteoporos Int, 2006. **17**(7): p. 1022-32.

666. Boskey, A.L., et al., *Effect of short-term hypomagnesemia on the chemical and mechanical properties of rat bone.* J Orthop Res, 1992. **10**(6): p. 774-83.

667. Kenney, M.A., H. McCoy, and L. Williams, *Effects of magnesium deficiency on strength, mass, and composition of rat femur.* Calcif Tissue Int, 1994. **54**(1): p. 44-9.

668. Matias, C.N., et al., *Magnesium intake mediates the association between bone mineral density and lean soft tissue in elite swimmers.* Magnes Res, 2012. **25**(3): p. 120-5.

669. Bertelloni, S., *The parathyroid hormone- 1,25-dihydroxyvitamin D endocrine system and magnesium status in insulin-dependent diabetes mellitus: current concepts.* Magnes Res, 1992. **5**(1): p. 45-51.

670. McNair, P., *Bone mineral metabolism in human type 1 (insulin dependent) diabetes mellitus.* Dan Med Bull, 1988. **35**(2): p. 109-21.

671. Saggese, G., et al., *Hypomagnesemia and the parathyroid hormone-vitamin D endocrine system in children with insulin-dependent diabetes mellitus: effects of magnesium administration.* J Pediatr, 1991. **118**(2): p. 220-5.

672. Aydin, H., et al., *Short-term oral magnesium supplementation suppresses bone turnover in postmenopausal osteoporotic women.* Biol Trace Elem Res, 2010. **133**(2): p. 136-43.

673. *Deoxypyridinoline (2023) Wikipedia. Available at: https://en.wikipedia.org/wiki/Deoxypyridinoline (Accessed: 06 July 2024).*

674. Stendig-Lindberg, G., R. Tepper, and I. Leichter, *Trabecular bone density in a two year controlled trial of peroral magnesium in osteoporosis.* Magnes Res, 1993. **6**(2): p. 155-63.

675. Dimai, H.P., et al., *Daily oral magnesium supplementation suppresses bone turnover in young adult males.* J Clin Endocrinol Metab, 1998. **83**(8): p. 2742-8.

676. Rondanelli, M., et al., *An update on magnesium and bone health.* Biometals, 2021. **34**(4): p. 715-736.

677. Carpenter, T.O., et al., *A randomized controlled study of effects of dietary magnesium oxide supplementation on bone mineral content in healthy girls.* J Clin Endocrinol Metab, 2006. **91**(12): p. 4866-72.

678. *Wood T, McKinnon T. Calcium-Magnesium-Vitamin D Supplementation Improves*

Bone Mineralization in Preadolescent Girls. 2001. USANA Clinical Research Bulletin, USANA Health Sciences, Inc. SLC, UT.

679. *How kidneys work (no date) Kidney Foundation. Available at: https://kidney.ca/Kidney-Health/Your-Kidneys/How-Kidneys-Work (Accessed: 16 July 2024).*

680. *Facts about chronic kidney disease (2024) National Kidney Foundation. Available at: https://www.kidney.org/atoz/content/about-chronic-kidney-disease (Accessed: 16 July 2024).*

681. Macías Ruiz, M.D.C., et al., *Magnesium in Kidney Function and Disease-Implications for Aging and Sex-A Narrative Review.* Nutrients, 2023. **15**(7).

682. Blaine, J., M. Chonchol, and M. Levi, *Renal control of calcium, phosphate, and magnesium homeostasis.* Clin J Am Soc Nephrol, 2015. **10**(7): p. 1257-72.

683. Rebholz, C.M., et al., *Dietary Magnesium and Kidney Function Decline: The Healthy Aging in Neighborhoods of Diversity across the Life Span Study.* Am J Nephrol, 2016. **44**(5): p. 381-387.

684. Vermeulen, E.A. and M.G. Vervloet, *Magnesium Administration in Chronic Kidney Disease.* Nutrients, 2023. **15**(3).

685. *What is chronic kidney disease? - niddk (no date) National Institute of Diabetes and Digestive and Kidney Diseases. Available at: https://www.niddk.nih.gov/health-information/kidney-disease/chronic-kidney-disease-ckd/what-is-chronic-kidney-disease (Accessed: 16 July 2024).*

686. Cunningham, J., M. Rodríguez, and P. Messa, *Magnesium in chronic kidney disease Stages 3 and 4 and in dialysis patients.* Clin Kidney J, 2012. **5**(Suppl 1): p. i39-i51.

687. Mountokalakis, T.D., *Magnesium metabolism in chronic renal failure.* Magnes Res, 1990. **3**(2): p. 121-7.

688. Curry, J.N. and A.S.L. Yu, *Magnesium Handling in the Kidney.* Adv Chronic Kidney Dis, 2018. **25**(3): p. 236-243.

689. Farhadnejad, H., et al., *Micronutrient Intakes and Incidence of Chronic Kidney Disease in Adults: Tehran Lipid and Glucose Study.* Nutrients, 2016. **8**(4): p. 217.

690. Maier, J.A., et al., *Low magnesium promotes endothelial cell dysfunction: implications for atherosclerosis, inflammation and thrombosis.* Biochim Biophys Acta, 2004. **1689**(1): p. 13-21.

691. Lacson, E., Jr., et al., *Serum Magnesium and Mortality in Hemodialysis Patients in the United States: A Cohort Study.* Am J Kidney Dis, 2015. **66**(6): p. 1056-66.

692. Van Laecke, S., et al., *Hypomagnesemia and the risk of death and GFR decline in chronic kidney disease.* Am J Med, 2013. **126**(9): p. 825-31.

693. Salem, S., et al., *Relationship between magnesium and clinical biomarkers on inhibition of vascular calcification.* Am J Nephrol, 2012. **35**(1): p. 31-9.

694. Workinger, J.L., R.P. Doyle, and J. Bortz, *Challenges in the Diagnosis of Magnesium Status.* Nutrients, 2018. **10**(9).

695. Moe, O.W., *Kidney stones: pathophysiology and medical management.* Lancet, 2006. **367**(9507): p. 333-44.

696. Wu, J., et al., *Association Between Serum Magnesium and the Prevalence of Kidney Stones: a Cross-sectional Study.* Biol Trace Elem Res, 2020. **195**(1): p. 20-26.

697. Pearle, M.S., et al., *Medical management of kidney stones: AUA guideline.* J Urol, 2014. **192**(2): p. 316-24.

698. Johansson, G., et al., *Effects of magnesium hydroxide in renal stone disease.* J Am Coll Nutr, 1982. **1**(2): p. 179-85.

699. Shringi, S., C.A. Raker, and J. Tang, *Dietary Magnesium Intake and Kidney Stone: The National Health and Nutrition Examination Survey 2011-2018.* R I Med J (2013), 2023. **106**(11): p. 20-25.

700. Voss, S., et al., *The effect of oral administration of calcium and magnesium on intestinal oxalate absorption in humans.* Isotopes Environ Health Stud, 2004. **40**(3): p. 199-205.

701. Riley, J.M., et al., *Effect of magnesium on calcium and oxalate ion binding.* J Endourol, 2013. **27**(12): p. 1487-92.

702. Reungjui, S., et al., *Magnesium status of patients with renal stones and its effect on urinary citrate excretion.* BJU Int, 2002. **90**(7): p. 635-9.

703. *Gates B Colbert, M. (2024) Hypocitraturia: Practice essentials, importance of citrate, risk factors in hypocitraturia, Hypocitraturia: Practice Essentials, Importance of Citrate, Risk Factors in Hypocitraturia. Available at: https://emedicine.medscape.com/article/444968-overview?form=fpf (Accessed: 18 July 2024).*

704. Koh, E.T., S. Reiser, and M. Fields, *Dietary fructose as compared to glucose and starch increases the calcium content of kidney of magnesium-deficient rats.* J Nutr, 1989. **119**(8): p. 1173-8.

705. Labeeuw, M., et al., *[Role of magnesium in the physiopathology and treatment of calcium renal lithiasis].* Presse Med, 1987. **16**(1): p. 25-7.

706. Eisner, B.H., et al., *High dietary magnesium intake decreases hyperoxaluria in patients with nephrolithiasis.* Urology, 2012. **80**(4): p. 780-3.

707. Kato, Y., et al., *Changes in urinary parameters after oral administration of potassium-sodium citrate and magnesium oxide to prevent urolithiasis.* Urology, 2004. **63**(1): p. 7-11; discussion 11-2.

708. Massey, L., *Magnesium therapy for nephrolithiasis.* Magnes Res, 2005. **18**(2): p. 123-6.

709. Micha, R., et al., *Association Between Dietary Factors and Mortality From Heart Disease, Stroke, and Type 2 Diabetes in the United States.* Jama, 2017. **317**(9): p. 912-924.

710. Thomas, D., *The mineral depletion of foods available to us as a nation (1940-2002)--a review of the 6th Edition of McCance and Widdowson.* Nutr Health, 2007. **19**(1-2): p. 21-55.

711. Mayer, A.B., L. Trenchard, and F. Rayns, *Historical changes in the mineral content of fruit and vegetables in the UK from 1940 to 2019: a concern for human nutrition and agriculture.* Int J Food Sci Nutr, 2022. **73**(3): p. 315-326.

712. *Davis DR. Declining Fruit and Vegetable Nutrient Composition: What is the Evidence. Hortscience. Vol. 44(1). February. 2009. .*

713. McCarty, M.F. and J.J. DiNicolantonio, *Acarbose, lente carbohydrate, and prebiotics promote metabolic health and longevity by stimulating intestinal production of GLP-1.* Open Heart, 2015. **2**(1): p. e000205.

714. DiNicolantonio, J.J. and A. Berger, *Added sugars drive nutrient and energy deficit in obesity: a new paradigm.* Open Heart, 2016. **3**(2): p. e000469.

715. Fiorentini, D., et al., *Magnesium: Biochemistry, Nutrition, Detection, and Social Impact of Diseases Linked to Its Deficiency.* Nutrients, 2021. **13**(4).

716. *Davis DR. Impact of Breeding and Yield on Fruit, Vegetable and Grain Nutrient Content.*

Breeding for Fruit Quality, First Edition. John Wiley & Sons, Inc. 2011.

717. *Guo W, Nazim H, Liang Z, et al.. Magnesium deficiency in plants: an urgent problem. Crop J 2016;4:83–91.*

718. Stover, P.J. and M.S. Field, *Vitamin B-6.* Adv Nutr, 2015. **6**(1): p. 132-3.

719. Lopes, A., et al., *Evaluation of the effects of fructose on oxidative stress and inflammatory parameters in rat brain.* Mol Neurobiol, 2014. **50**(3): p. 1124-30.

720. Delbosc, S., et al., *Involvement of oxidative stress and NADPH oxidase activation in the development of cardiovascular complications in a model of insulin resistance, the fructose-fed rat.* Atherosclerosis, 2005. **179**(1): p. 43-9.

721. Stanhope, K.L., et al., *Consuming fructose-sweetened, not glucose-sweetened, beverages increases visceral adiposity and lipids and decreases insulin sensitivity in overweight/obese humans.* J Clin Invest, 2009. **119**(5): p. 1322-34.

722. Lorincz, C., S.L. Manske, and R. Zernicke, *Bone health: part 1, nutrition.* Sports Health, 2009. **1**(3): p. 253-60.

723. DiNicolantonio, J.J. and S.C. Lucan, *Is fructose malabsorption a cause of irritable bowel syndrome?* Med Hypotheses, 2015. **85**(3): p. 295-7.

724. Ivaturi, R. and C. Kies, *Mineral balances in humans as affected by fructose, high fructose corn syrup and sucrose.* Plant Foods Hum Nutr, 1992. **42**(2): p. 143-51.

725. Shapiro, A., et al., *Fructose-induced leptin resistance exacerbates weight gain in response to subsequent high-fat feeding.* Am J Physiol Regul Integr Comp Physiol, 2008. **295**(5): p. R1370-5.

726. Huby, A.C., et al., *Adipocyte-Derived Hormone Leptin Is a Direct Regulator of Aldosterone Secretion, Which Promotes Endothelial Dysfunction and Cardiac Fibrosis.* Circulation, 2015. **132**(22): p. 2134-45.

727. *DiNicolantonio JJ. The Salt Fix. Harmony. 2017. https://www.penguinrandomhouse.com/books/545379/the-salt-fix-by-dr-james-dinicolantonio/9780451496966/.*

728. Nishimuta, M., et al., *Positive correlation between dietary intake of sodium and balances of calcium and magnesium in young Japanese adults--low sodium intake is a risk factor for loss of calcium and magnesium.* J Nutr Sci Vitaminol (Tokyo), 2005. **51**(4): p. 265-70.

729. Nishimuta, M., et al., *Equilibrium intakes of calcium and magnesium within an adequate and limited range of sodium intake in human.* J Nutr Sci Vitaminol (Tokyo), 2006. **52**(6): p. 402-6.

730. Brink, E.J., et al., *Interaction of calcium and phosphate decreases ileal magnesium solubility and apparent magnesium absorption in rats.* J Nutr, 1992. **122**(3): p. 580-6.

731. Lemann, J., Jr., et al., *Evidence that glucose ingestion inhibits net renal tubular reabsorption of calcium and magnesium in man.* J Lab Clin Med, 1970. **75**(4): p. 578-85.

732. Holl, M.G. and L.H. Allen, *Sucrose ingestion, insulin response and mineral metabolism in humans.* J Nutr, 1987. **117**(7): p. 1229-33.

733. Jones, J.E., R. Schwartz, and L. Krook, *Calcium homeostasis and bone pathology in magnesium deficient rats.* Calcif Tissue Int, 1980. **31**(3): p. 231-8.

734. Lennon, E.J., et al., *The effect of glucose on urinary cation excretion during chronic extracellular volume expansion in normal man.* J Clin Invest, 1974. **53**(5): p. 1424-33.

735. O'Dell, B.L., *Magnesium requirement and its relation to other dietary constituents.* Fed Proc, 1960. **19**: p. 648-54.

736. Bunce, G.E., et al., *DIETARY PHOSPHORUS AND MAGNESIUM DEFICIENCY IN THE RAT.* J Nutr, 1965. **86**: p. 406-13.

737. Bunce, G.E., Y. Chiemchaisri, and P.H. Phillips, *The mineral requirements of the dog. IV. Effect of certain dietary and physiologic factors upon the magnesium deficiency syndrome.* J Nutr, 1962. **76**(1): p. 23-9.

738. *Self Nutrition Data. Nutrition facts label for Cheese, cheddar.* http:// nutritiondata.self.com/facts/dairy-and-egg-products/8/2.

739. Gröber, U., J. Schmidt, and K. Kisters, *Magnesium in Prevention and Therapy.* Nutrients, 2015. **7**(9): p. 8199-226.

740. Neathery, M.W., et al., *Effects of dietary aluminum and phosphorus on magnesium metabolism in dairy calves.* J Anim Sci, 1990. **68**(4): p. 1133-8.

741. Hoorn, E.J. and R. Zietse, *Disorders of calcium and magnesium balance: a physiology-based approach.* Pediatr Nephrol, 2013. **28**(8): p. 1195-206.

742. Schlingmann, K.P., et al., *TRPM6 and TRPM7--Gatekeepers of human magnesium metabolism.* Biochim Biophys Acta, 2007. **1772**(8): p. 813-21.

743. Uribarri, J. and M.S. Calvo, *Hidden sources of phosphorus in the typical American diet: does it matter in nephrology?* Semin Dial, 2003. **16**(3): p. 186-8.

744. Norman, D.A., et al., *Jejunal and ileal adaptation to alterations in dietary calcium: changes in calcium and magnesium absorption and pathogenetic role of parathyroid hormone and 1,25-dihydroxyvitamin D.* J Clin Invest, 1981. **67**(6): p. 1599-603.

745. Hardwick, L.L., et al., *Magnesium absorption: mechanisms and the influence of vitamin D, calcium and phosphate.* J Nutr, 1991. **121**(1): p. 13-23.

746. Krejs, G.J., et al., *Effect of 1,25-dihydroxyvitamin D3 on calcium and magnesium absorption in the healthy human jejunum and ileum.* Am J Med, 1983. **75**(6): p. 973-6.

747. Hodgkinson, A., D.H. Marshall, and B.E. Nordin, *Vitamin D and magnesium absorption in man.* Clin Sci (Lond), 1979. **57**(1): p. 121-3.

748. Levine, B.S., et al., *Effects of vitamin D and diet magnesium on magnesium metabolism.* Am J Physiol, 1980. **239**(6): p. E515-23.

749. Scharf, E., et al., *The Effects of Prolonged Water-Only Fasting and Refeeding on Markers of Cardiometabolic Risk.* Nutrients, 2022. **14**(6).

750. Trepanowski, J.F. and R.J. Bloomer, *The impact of religious fasting on human health.* Nutr J, 2010. **9**: p. 57.

751. Wang, Y. and R. Wu, *The Effect of Fasting on Human Metabolism and Psychological Health.* Dis Markers, 2022. **2022**: p. 5653739.

752. Mehanna, H.M., J. Moledina, and J. Travis, *Refeeding syndrome: what it is, and how to prevent and treat it.* Bmj, 2008. **336**(7659): p. 1495-8.

753. Stewart, W.K. and L.W. Fleming, *Relationship between plasma and erythrocyte magnesium and potassium concentrations in fasting obese subjects.* Metabolism, 1973. **22**(4): p. 535-47.

754. Stewart, W.K. and L.W. Fleming, *Features of a successful therapeutic fast of 382 days' duration.* Postgrad Med J, 1973. **49**(569): p. 203-9.

755. Seelig, M.S., *Magnesium requirements in human nutrition.* J Med Soc N J, 1982. **79**(11): p. 849-50.

756. Durlach, J., et al., *Cardiovasoprotective foods and nutrients: possible importance of magnesium intake.* Magnes Res, 1999. **12**(1): p. 57-61.

757. *Office of dietary supplements - thiamin (no date) NIH Office of Dietary Supplements. Available at: https://ods.od.nih.gov/factsheets/Thiamin-HealthProfessional/ (Accessed: 14 August 2024).*

758. *Eby GA, Eby KL, Murk H. Magnesium and major depression. In: Vink R, Nechifor M, editors. Magnesium in the Central Nervous System [Internet]. Adelaide (AU): University of Adelaide Press; 2011. Available from: https://www.ncbi.nlm.nih.gov/books/NBK507265/#.*

759. van den Heuvel, E.G., et al., *Short-chain fructo-oligosaccharides improve magnesium absorption in adolescent girls with a low calcium intake.* Nutr Res, 2009. **29**(4): p. 229-37.

760. Kolte, D., et al., *Role of magnesium in cardiovascular diseases.* Cardiol Rev, 2014. **22**(4): p. 182-92.

761. *https://health.clevelandclinic.org/foods-that-are-high-in-magnesium.*

762. *Office of dietary supplements - magnesium (no date) NIH Office of Dietary Supplements. Available at: https://ods.od.nih.gov/factsheets/Magnesium-HealthProfessional/ (Accessed: 23 August 2024).*

763. Ates, M., et al., *Dose-Dependent Absorption Profile of Different Magnesium Compounds.* Biol Trace Elem Res, 2019. **192**(2): p. 244-251.

764. *National Center for Biotechnology Information (2024). PubChem Compound Summary for CID 73981, Magnesium Hydroxide. Retrieved August 26, 2024 from https://pubchem.ncbi.nlm.nih.gov/compound/Magnesium-Hydroxide.*

765. *Hanusa, T. P. (2024, August 2). magnesium. Encyclopedia Britannica. https://www.britannica.com/science/magnesium.*

766. Garg, V., P. Narang, and R. Taneja, *Antacids revisited: review on contemporary facts and relevance for self-management.* J Int Med Res, 2022. **50**(3): p. 3000605221086457.

767. *https://reference.medscape.com/drug/milk-of-magnesia-magnesium-hydroxide-342018.*

768. Tedesco, F.J. and J.T. DiPiro, *Laxative use in constipation. American College of Gastroenterology's Committee on FDA-Related Matters.* Am J Gastroenterol, 1985. **80**(4): p. 303-9.

769. *Magnesium hydroxide (2024) Wikipedia. Available at: https://en.wikipedia.org/wiki/Magnesium_hydroxide#cite_note-10 (Accessed: 26 August 2024).*

770. *What is magnesium hydroxide used for? (no date) Synapse. Available at: https://synapse.patsnap.com/article/what-is-magnesium-hydroxide-used-for (Accessed: 26 August 2024).*

771. Hutchison, A.J. and M. Wilkie, *Use of magnesium as a drug in chronic kidney disease.* Clin Kidney J, 2012. **5**(Suppl 1): p. i62-i70.

772. Mori, H., J. Tack, and H. Suzuki, *Magnesium Oxide in Constipation.* Nutrients, 2021. **13**(2).

773. Fukushima, S., et al., *A Study on the Safety of Long-Term Magnesium Oxide Administration in Elderly Patients with Impaired Renal Function.* 医薬品情報学, 2021. **23**(3): p. 129-134.

774. Mori, S., et al., *A Randomized Double-blind Placebo-controlled Trial on the Effect of Magnesium Oxide in Patients With Chronic Constipation.* J Neurogastroenterol Motil, 2019. **25**(4): p. 563-575.

775. Firoz, M. and M. Graber, *Bioavailability of US commercial magnesium preparations.* Magnes Res, 2001. **14**(4): p. 257-62.

776. Ranade, V.V. and J.C. Somberg, *Bioavailability and pharmacokinetics of magnesium after administration of magnesium salts to humans.* Am J Ther, 2001. **8**(5): p. 345-57.

777. Rodríguez-Moran, M. and F. Guerrero-Romero, *Oral magnesium supplementation improves the metabolic profile of metabolically obese, normal-weight individuals: a randomized double-blind placebo-controlled trial.* Arch Med Res, 2014. **45**(5): p. 388-93.

778. Simental-Mendía, L.E., M. Rodríguez-Morán, and F. Guerrero-Romero, *Oral magnesium supplementation decreases C-reactive protein levels in subjects with prediabetes and hypomagnesemia: a clinical randomized double-blind placebo-controlled trial.* Arch Med Res, 2014. **45**(4): p. 325-30.

779. Gröber, U., et al., *Myth or Reality-Transdermal Magnesium?* Nutrients, 2017. **9**(8).

780. Landeras, L.A., R. Aslam, and J. Yee, *Virtual colonoscopy: technique and accuracy.* Radiol Clin North Am, 2007. **45**(2): p. 333-45.

781. *Magnesium citrate: Health benefits, nutrients per serving, preparation information, and more (no date a) WebMD. Available at: https://www.webmd.com/diet/health-benefits-magnesium-citrate (Accessed: 29 August 2024).*

782. Köseoglu, E., et al., *The effects of magnesium prophylaxis in migraine without aura.* Magnes Res, 2008. **21**(2): p. 101-8.

783. Mah, J. and T. Pitre, *Oral magnesium supplementation for insomnia in older adults: a Systematic Review & Meta-Analysis.* BMC Complement Med Ther, 2021. **21**(1): p. 125.

784. Gorantla, S., A. Ravisankar, and L.M. Trotti, *Magnesium citrate monotherapy improves restless legs syndrome symptoms and multiple suggested immobilization test scores in an open-label pilot study.* J Clin Sleep Med, 2024. **20**(8): p. 1357-1361.

785. Spasov, A.A., et al., *[Comparative study of magnesium salts bioavailability in rats fed a magnesium-deficient diet].* Vestn Ross Akad Med Nauk, 2010(2): p. 29-37.

786. *NAGLE, F. J., BALKE, B., GANSLEN, R. V., & DAVIS, A. W., Jr (1963). THE MITIGATION OF PHYSICAL FATIGUE WITH "SPARTASE". REP 63-12. [Report].* Civil Aeromedical Research Institute (U.S.).

787. *Magnesium glycinate (2024) Wikipedia.* Available at: https://en.wikipedia.org/wiki/Magnesium_glycinate (Accessed: 30 August 2024).

788. Uberti, F., et al., *Study of Magnesium Formulations on Intestinal Cells to Influence Myometrium Cell Relaxation.* Nutrients, 2020. **12**(2).

789. Razak, M.A., et al., *Multifarious Beneficial Effect of Nonessential Amino Acid, Glycine: A Review.* Oxid Med Cell Longev, 2017. **2017**: p. 1716701.

790. Supakatisant, C. and V. Phupong, *Oral magnesium for relief in pregnancy-induced leg cramps: a randomised controlled trial.* Matern Child Nutr, 2015. **11**(2): p. 139-45.

791. Schaffer, S.W., et al., *Physiological roles of taurine in heart and muscle.* J Biomed Sci, 2010. **17 Suppl 1**(Suppl 1): p. S2.

792. McCarty, M.F., *Complementary vascular-protective actions of magnesium and taurine: a rationale for magnesium taurate.* Med Hypotheses, 1996. **46**(2): p. 89-100.

793. Shrivastava, P., et al., *Magnesium taurate attenuates progression of hypertension and cardiotoxicity against cadmium chloride-induced hypertensive albino rats.* J Tradit Complement Med, 2019. **9**(2): p. 119-123.

794. *Huda Latif Hasan, & Maysaa Jalal Majeed. (2024). The Promising Role of Magnesium Taurate in Managing Hypertension. Modern Sport, 23(1), 0134-0142.* https://doi.org/10.54702/vjwzc706.

795. McCarty, M.F., *Magnesium taurate for the prevention and treatment of pre-eclampsia/eclampsia.* Med Hypotheses, 1996. **47**(4): p. 269-72.

796. Uysal, N., et al., *Timeline (Bioavailability) of Magnesium Compounds in Hours: Which Magnesium Compound Works Best?* Biol Trace Elem Res, 2019. **187**(1): p. 128-136.

797. Hosgorler, F., et al., *Magnesium Acetyl Taurate Prevents Tissue Damage and Deterioration of Prosocial Behavior Related with Vasopressin Levels in Traumatic Brain Injured Rats.* Turk Neurosurg, 2020. **30**(5): p. 723-733.

798. *Haddad A, Mohiuddin SS. Biochemistry, Citric Acid Cycle. [Updated 2023 May 1]. In: StatPearls [Internet]. Treasure Island (FL): StatPearls Publishing; 2024 Jan-. Available from:* https://www.ncbi.nlm.nih.gov/books/NBK541072/#.

799. de Carvalho, J.F. and A. Lerner, *Malic Acid for the Treatment of Rheumatic Diseases.* Mediterr J Rheumatol, 2023. **34**(4): p. 592-593.

800. Russell, I.J., et al., *Treatment of fibromyalgia syndrome with Super Malic: a randomized, double blind, placebo controlled, crossover pilot study.* J Rheumatol, 1995. **22**(5): p. 953-8.

801. *Abraham, G. E., & Flechas, J. D. (1992). Management of Fibromyalgia: Rationale for the Use of Magnesium and Malic Acid. Journal of Nutritional Medicine, 3(1), 49–59.* https://doi.org/10.3109/13590849208997961.

802. *Sapra A, Bhandari P. Chronic Fatigue Syndrome. [Updated 2023 Jun 21]. In: StatPearls [Internet]. Treasure Island (FL): StatPearls Publishing; 2024 Jan-. Available from:* https://www.ncbi.nlm.nih.gov/books/NBK557676/.

803. Zhang, Y., et al., *Can Magnesium Enhance Exercise Performance?* Nutrients, 2017. **9**(9).

804. Zeana, C., *Magnesium orotate in myocardial and neuronal protection.* Rom J Intern Med, 1999. **37**(1): p. 91-7.

805. Classen, H.G., *Magnesium orotate--experimental and clinical evidence.* Rom J Intern Med, 2004. **42**(3): p. 491-501.

806. Stepura, O.B., F.E. Tomaeva, and T.V. Zvereva, *[Orotic acid as a metabolic agent].* Vestn Ross Akad Med Nauk, 2002(2): p. 39-41.

807. Branea, I., et al., *Assessment of treatment with orotate magnesium in early postoperative period of patients with cardiac insufficiency and coronary artery by-pass grafts (ATOMIC).* Rom J Intern Med, 1999. **37**(3): p. 287-96.

808. Geiss, K.R., et al., *Effects of magnesium orotate on exercise tolerance in patients with coronary heart disease.* Cardiovasc Drugs Ther, 1998. **12 Suppl 2**: p. 153-6.

809. Golf, S.W., S. Bender, and J. Grüttner, *On the significance of magnesium in extreme physical stress.* Cardiovasc Drugs Ther, 1998. **12 Suppl 2**: p. 197-202.

810. McCarty, M.F. and J.J. DiNicolantonio, *β-Alanine and orotate as supplements for cardiac protection.* Open Heart, 2014. **1**(1): p. e000119.

811. Schiopu, C., et al., *Magnesium Orotate and the Microbiome-Gut-Brain Axis Modulation: New Approaches in Psychological Comorbidities of Gastrointestinal Functional Disorders.* Nutrients, 2022. **14**(8).

812. Sun, Q., et al., *Regulation of structural and functional synapse density by L-threonate through modulation of intraneuronal magnesium concentration.* Neuropharmacology, 2016. **108**: p. 426-39.

813. Scheff, S.W. and D.A. Price, *Alzheimer's disease-related alterations in synaptic density: neocortex and hippocampus.* J Alzheimers Dis, 2006. **9**(3 Suppl): p. 101-15.

814. Slutsky, I., et al., *Enhancement of learning and memory by elevating brain magnesium.* Neuron, 2010. **65**(2): p. 165-77.

815. Li, W., et al., *Elevation of brain magnesium prevents synaptic loss and reverses cognitive deficits in Alzheimer's disease mouse model.* Mol Brain, 2014. **7**: p. 65.

816. Liu, G., et al., *Efficacy and Safety of MMFS-01, a Synapse Density Enhancer, for Treating Cognitive Impairment in Older Adults: A Randomized, Double-Blind, Placebo-Controlled Trial.* J Alzheimers Dis, 2016. **49**(4): p. 971-90.

817. Wroolie, T.E., et al., *An 8-week open label trial of L-Threonic Acid Magnesium Salt in patients with mild to moderate dementia.* Personalized medicine in psychiatry., 2017. **4-6**: p. 7-12.

818. Kowalski, K. and A. Mulak, *Brain-Gut-Microbiota Axis in Alzheimer's Disease.* J Neurogastroenterol Motil, 2019. **25**(1): p. 48-60.

819. Liao, W., et al., *Magnesium-L-threonate treats Alzheimer's disease by modulating the microbiota-gut-brain axis.* Neural Regen Res, 2024. **19**(10): p. 2281-2289.

820. Surman, C., et al., *L-Threonic Acid Magnesium Salt Supplementation in ADHD: An Open-Label Pilot Study.* J Diet Suppl, 2021. **18**(2): p. 119-131.

821. Lu, J.F. and C.H. Nightingale, *Magnesium sulfate in eclampsia and pre-eclampsia: pharmacokinetic principles.* Clin Pharmacokinet, 2000. **38**(4): p. 305-14.

822. Hoffer, M., et al., *Utility of magnesium sulfate in the treatment of rapid atrial fibrillation in the emergency department: a systematic review and meta-analysis.* Eur J Emerg Med, 2022. **29**(4): p. 253-261.

823. *Dinesh Chandra Damor, Jitendra Pujari, M.U Mansuri, Vijay Singh Rawat. A comparative study to assess the effectiveness of Epsom salt with hot water versus plain water on pain and*

functional performance among arthritis patients at selected hospital, Udaipur. Int J Health Sci Res. 2023;13(9):137-149. DOI: 10.52403/ijhsr.20230921.

Made in the USA
Las Vegas, NV
02 October 2024

96143328R00138